MIGRAINE
QUESTIONS AND ANSWERS

SECOND EDITION

Egilius L.H. Spierings, M.D, Ph.D.
Associate Clinical Professor, Department of Neurology
Brigham and Women's Hospital, Harvard Medical School,
Boston, Massachusetts

Dedicated to my children, Sven and Natalia, the pride of my life

me rit
PUBLISHING
INTERNATIONAL

me**e**rit

PUBLISHING
INTERNATIONAL

MIGRAINE

QUESTIONS AND ANSWERS

SECOND EDITION

MERIT PUBLISHING INTERNATIONAL

European address:
35 Winchester Street
Basingstoke
Hampshire RG21 7EE
England
Tel: (+44)1256 841008
Fax: (+44)1256 841099
e-mail: merituk@aol.com

North American address:
5840 Corporate Way
Suite 200
West Palm Beach, FL 33407
U.S.A.
Tel: (561)697 1116
Fax: (561)477 4961
e-mail: meritpi@aol.com

Web: www.meritpublishing.com

ISBN: 1 873413 96 3

Egilius L.H. Spierings, M.D, Ph.D.

me rit
PUBLISHING
INTERNATIONAL

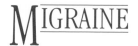

CONTENTS

The successful treatment of migraine is difficult but worth the effort. It taps every resource of the physician. Probably more hours of suffering are caused by migraine than by any other human affliction. Knowledge of its secrets is incomplete but increasing. For these reasons it presents a unique challenge.

John R. Graham, M.D., M.A.C.P.*

4

FOREWORD

Headache is one of the most common complaints of mankind and almost everyone knows what it is like to have one. Taking over-the-counter medications from the dizzying array available in the pharmacy treats most headaches. However, many people eventually seek the help of a physician, particularly if the headaches are frequent or intense, or when they frighten the headache sufferer by raising the specter of serious neurological illness, in particularly brain tumor. The sheer number of people suffering from headache makes it one of the most common reasons for which medical attention is sought; it is the most common reason that a neurological consultation is pursued.

Fortunately, the number of people presenting with headache who are found to have a serious underlying neurological illness is few, leaving a vast number, of whom the majority have migraine or related headache types. Many of these patients drift from doctor to doctor, episodically visit emergency departments, seek alternative treatments, become alienated from the medical profession, and often never improve or even worsen, owing to the complex interaction between headache, environmental factors, and various drug treatments. Some develop difficulties related to opioid use and are a source of untold frustration for medical care providers, their families, and, most importantly, themselves.

The irony is that given modern knowledge about the pathophysiology and pharmacology of migraine, much can be done to help the huge number of people and often prevent the bad outcomes. In this book on Migraine, Egilius L.H. Spierings shares his enormous experience in the treatment of this common medical condition. Using a case-based question-and-answer method, he gives us a tried and true method for handling migraine and related

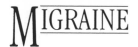
MIGRAINE

disorders, so that we can avoid iatrogenic worsening of the patient's condition and still provide significant and often dramatic relief.

This book should provide the general medical practitioner, internist, or pediatrician with the necessary knowledge to manage the vast majority of patients with headache problems, dramatically reducing the prevalence of iatrogenic complications, as well as the need for neurological consultation. Dr. Spierings' book may not, in actual fact, reduce the prevalence of migraine but could dramatically reduce the suffering it causes to all of us.

Martin A. Samuels, M.D.
Chairman of Neurology, Brigham and Women's Hospital
Professor of Neurology, Harvard Medical School

CHAPTER 1

INTRODUCTION

What is this book about?

This book is about migraine, one of the most common conditions of mankind, known to us through writings since 3,000 BC. Migraine affects, with greater or lesser regularity and throughout much of their lifetime, an estimated 10-15% of the population. It causes disability, be it often temporary, and strains personal relationships and professional development. Nevertheless, little is known about it in scientific terms and, hence, its treatment remains mostly empirical; it is, therefore, the clinician who carries the flag and directs the path for research to follow.

Through a system of questions and answers, this book covers the topic of migraine conditions. The chapters are written in such a way that they can be read and understood individually, without reference to previous chapters. The material is presented at the level of the primary-care physician, with emphasis on the clinical aspects. However, the book also provides good and clear reading for the educated migraine patient. The material is illustrated, wherever possible, with case studies based on actual patients the author has cared for.

After defining and classifying migraine, the epidemiology of the condition is reviewed, followed by a discussion of its symptomatology, pathogenesis, and diagnosis. Abortive and preventive treatment as well as the migraine trigger factors are discussed in three separate chapters. Words of wisdom from my mentor in headache management for the patients with migraine and their physicians concludes the book.

Who is the author?

The author, Dr. Spierings, a native of The Netherlands, currently lives in the United States. He received his M.D.-degree from the Medical Faculty of the Erasmus University in Rotterdam, The Netherlands, in 1978 and received his Ph.D.-degree in experimental pharmacology from the same university in 1980. He was an intern in neurosurgery in 1980-81 and a fellow in headache management with John Ruskin Graham, M.D., M.A.C.P. at The Headache Research Foundation in Boston, Massachusetts, in 1981-82. From 1982 until 1985, Dr. Spierings was a resident in neurology at the University Hospital "Dijkzigt" in Rotterdam and in 1985 he was a resident in psychiatry at the Hippolytus Hospital in Delft, The Netherlands.

In 1986, Dr. Spierings was appointed director of The Headache Research Foundation in Boston where, in 1987, he founded the John R. Graham Headache Centre. From 1990 until 1994, Dr. Spierings was the director of the Headache Section of the Division of Neurology at Brigham and Women's Hospital in Boston. In 1994, he set up a private practice dedicated to headache in Wellesley Hills, Massachusetts. He has remained affiliated with Brigham and Women's Hospital as a consultant in neurology. In 1996, he co-founded the Boston Clinical Research Center in Wellesley Hills, a center for clinical-trial research.

From 1986 until 1990, Dr. Spierings was an assistant professor of neurology at Tufts University School of Medicine in Boston. He has been affiliated with Harvard Medical School since where he is presently an associate clinical professor of neurology. He is a fellow of the American Headache Society, formerly known as American Association for the Study of Headache. He has published approximately 200 articles, reviews, and book chapters, authored seven books, and edited two monographs and three symposium proceedings. He is also the editor of the section on headache and pain of the textbook, *Office Practice of Neurology*. He has presented more than 600 lectures, posters, and workshops on headache and migraine throughout Europe, North and South America, and Australia. He organized sixteen symposia and two headache/migraine art exhibitions for The Headache Research Foundation, American Association for the Study of Headache, Headache Cooperative of New England, and Harvard Medical School.

Dr. Spierings is a former board member of the American Association for the Study of Headache and the International Headache Society. He is also a former associate editor of Cephalalgia, the journal of the International Headache Society. He is a founding member and the education director of the Headache Cooperative of New England. He has appeared in several biographies, including Who's Who Among Rising Young Americans, Men of Achievement, Who's Who in America, and Who's Who in the World.

Dr. Spierings was also listed in the 1994-95 Edition of The Best Doctors in America.

CHAPTER 2

DEFINITION

What is migraine?

Migraine is a chronic paroxysmal disorder with freedom from symptoms
in between the attacks. The attacks are stereotypical in their occurrence
and consist of transient focal neurological symptoms, headache, or both.
The transient focal neurological symptoms are almost always sensory in
nature, generally visual and sometimes somatosensory. The headache is
generally so intense that it interferes with the ability to function and can
be incapacitating to the extent that it requires bed rest. It is also of such
intensity that it interferes with the functioning of other systems in the
body. As a result, it often comes associated with other symptoms, such as
anorexia, nausea, photophobia, and phonophobia. Sometimes the
headache is also associated with osmophobia, blurred vision, vomiting, or
diarrhea. In addition, the patient tends to look pale and feel cold,
especially in the hands and feet.

The associated symptoms generally follow the onset of the headache and
increase in intensity as the headache increases in intensity. The
gastrointestinal symptoms progress from anorexia to nausea to vomiting
and the sensory symptoms from photophobia to phonophobia to
osmophobia. The transient focal neurological symptoms, on the other
hand, almost always precede the onset of the headache or occur during
the initial phase of headache development. For this reason they are
referred to as aura symptoms, which is the term that will be employed
throughout this text.

The attacks of migraine generally last less than one hour when merely
consisting of transient focal neurological symptoms but last for hours or
days when also headache is present. When the transient focal neurological
symptoms occur by themselves and without headache, the condition is
referred to as *isolated migraine aura* or *migraine aura without headache*.
It is referred to as *classic migraine or migraine with aura* when both the
transient focal neurological symptoms and headache occur. When the

headache occurs by itself, the condition is referred to as *common migraine* or *migraine without aura.*

Like many if not most medical conditions, there is a hereditary component to migraine, manifesting itself in a positive family history. It has been shown that migraine occurs in first-degree relatives in 60-70% of patients[3]. The risk of developing the condition is 45% when one parent is affected and 70% when both parents have migraine. It has been estimated that one-third of migraine expression is accounted for by genetic factors. The onset of the condition is almost always in the first three decades of life, often in the teenage or adolescent years. Unfortunately, for many of those afflicted, it is a life-long condition although the headaches may abate, especially in intensity, with the advancement of age.

The frequency with which the attacks of migraine occur varies tremendously: it can be as low as once per year or as high as once or twice per week. The frequency varies not only between individuals but also between periods of time within the same individual. However, on the average, migraine attacks occur once or twice per month, in women typically related to the menstrual cycle, that is, with menstruation and, to a lesser extent, with ovulation. With frequently occurring migraine headaches, so-called interval headaches of lesser intensity often occur in between the severe headaches. Interval headaches are also migraine headaches – although they may look like tension headaches – and abortively respond to specific antimigraine medications, including the triptans[2]. Ultimately, the migraine and interval headaches may merge into a daily headache condition, referred to as *chronic migraine*. It is also referred to as *transformed migraine*, in particular when the daily headaches developed out of (episodic) migraine headaches.

The variation in frequency of the attacks is related to the sensitivity of the condition to many endogenous and exogenous factors, referred to as trigger factors. A very potent endogenous trigger of migraine is the estrogen cycle in women, which largely accounts for the two or three times higher prevalence of migraine in women than in men. It may be the most potent trigger of migraine headaches, accounting for the onset of migraine in the early teens (menarche), the occurrence of attacks in relation to the menstrual cycle, the improvement during pregnancy, and the cessation of the condition with menopause.

How does migraine relate to other headache conditions?

Migraine is part of what I have referred to as the *vascular–headache spectrum* (Figure 2.1). The spectrum also includes jabs and jolts, paroxysmal hemicrania, and cluster headache. Jabs and jolts – also called stabbing headaches – are severe, sharp pains in the head, which last for seconds. They occur by themselves, as in the jabs and jolts syndrome, or in association with other vascular headaches, such as migraine or cluster headache. Their frequency varies greatly and ranges from once per month or less to several hundred times per day.

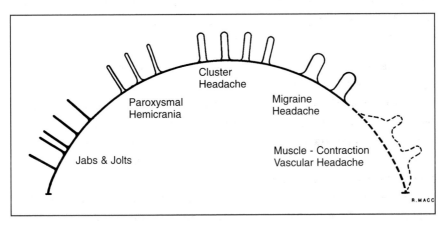

Figure 2.1. *The vascular-headache spectrum, including jabs and jolts, paroxysmal hemicrania, cluster headache, and migraine headache. Tension-type vascular headache is not a purely vascular headache condition; it forms the bridge between migraine and tension-type headache in the so-called tension-migraine headache continuum.*

Case study of jabs and jolts

A 53-year-old man has experienced headaches in the form of facial pains since age 25. The headaches consist of sharp jabs of pain, radiating from the right, first upper incisor into the cheek and eye. The jabs last for 5-30 seconds and many of them occur during the day. They are daily for several weeks at a time, separated by periods of three to four months without pain. The jabs either occur spontaneously or are precipitated by touching or biting down on the incisor or by brushing the teeth, shaving, eating, talking, coughing, *etc.* A root-canal procedure performed on the involved tooth failed to provide relief, as did anesthetic infiltration of the right infraorbital nerve. However, treatment with the combination of phenytoin, 100 mg, and diphenhydramine, 25 mg three times daily, helped to some extent. Subsequently, he was treated with carbamazepine, which provided control of the jabs. However, it required a dose as high as 1,200 mg per day, which caused considerable drowsiness.

At age 43, he underwent a radiofrequency procedure of the right trigeminal ganglion, which entirely eliminated the jabs for nine years. Then, the jabs returned as before and on a single day, he counted as many as 370! At the time of consultation, they occurred every 5-10 minutes for several consecutive hours at a time. Occasionally, when a jab hit him, he would cry out or jerk his head. He had almost completely stopped eating solid foods and now also drinking triggered the jabs. As a result, he had lost seven to eight pounds during the month prior to consultation. He was prescribed indomethacin, 75 mg (sustained release) twice daily, which decreased the frequency of the jabs to five or less per day.

Paroxysmal hemicrania is a variant of cluster headache with headaches lasting for 10-30 minutes and occurring five to fifteen times per day. Cluster headache is characterized by severe, unilateral headaches, usually located behind one eye, which last for 30 minutes to two hours. The headaches occur less frequently than in paroxysmal hemicrania, that is, once or twice per day, and typically occur at night, waking the patient up out of sleep between midnight and 2a.m.

The vascular headaches respond, abortively as well as preventively, to vasoconstrictors, such as ergots and triptans. The shorter-lasting vascular headaches, that is, jabs and jolts and paroxysmal hemicrania, also respond preventively to treatment with indomethacin, a non-steroidal anti-inflammatory medication. Paroxysmal hemicrania and cluster headache, like the predominantly nocturnally occurring headaches in general, can also be treated effectively with a calcium-entry blocker, such as verapamil.

How does migraine relate to ordinary headache?

The International Headache Society refers to ordinary, stress or tension headache as episodic tension-type headache. It is a headache that is ubiquitously experienced, affecting 63% of men and 86% of women[4]. It is mild or moderate in intensity and does not interfere with the ability to function or with the functioning of other systems in the body. It is, therefore, generally not associated with other symptoms, except for occasional mild photophobia or phonophobia. It tends to be bilateral in location, across the forehead, on top, or in the back of the head. It typically comes on in the late afternoon and is relieved by a non-prescription analgesic, rest, or relaxation.

How does migraine affect the quality of life?

Although free from migraine symptoms in between the attacks, the patients are not free from symptoms altogether and, as a result, experience decreased well-being. This was shown in a study of 138 migraine patients who were compared with a random population sample, equal in size and matched in age and gender[1]. The questionnaires applied were the Subjective Symptoms Assessment Profile and Psychological General Well-being Index. The questionnaires inquired about symptoms and affective states experienced during the preceding month. The symptoms were categorized into the six dimensions of emotional distress, gastrointestinal symptoms, peripheral vascular symptoms, cardiac symptoms, sex life, and dizziness. The patients scored significantly worse

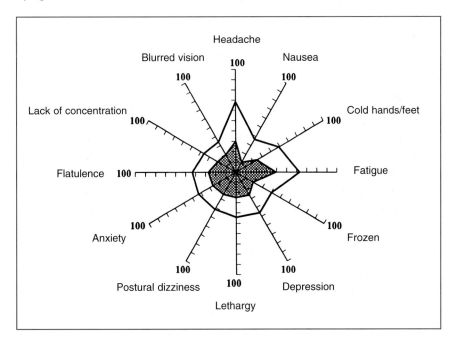

Figure 2.2. *The 12 items of the Subjective Symptoms Assessment Profile that migraine patients (n = 138; open area) scored worst on, in comparison to age- and gender-matched controls (n = 138; shaded area). Reproduced from reference 1.*

on all six dimensions, in particular on those of emotional distress and gastrointestinal symptoms. The symptoms that were worst in the migraine patients, in comparison to the non-headache controls, are shown in Figure 2.2. The five symptoms that most distinguished the two groups were headache, nausea, cold hands/feet, fatigue, and feeling cold (frozen). The latter three symptoms, that is, fatigue, feeling cold, and cold hands/feet, may reflect a lower energy metabolism in the patients[5].

With regard to the affective states, also categorized into six dimensions, the migraine patients scored worse on all of them as well, in comparison to the controls (Figure 2.3). However, they scored particularly poorly on the dimensions of anxiety and vitality: the average shift was calculated to be 5-10%, which was considered to be of moderate clinical significance. However, more importantly than being of clinical significance, the anxiety and lack of vitality may affect the ability of the patients to function on a daily basis and enjoy life.

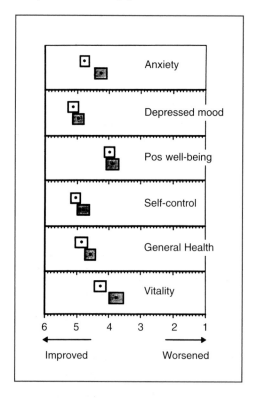

Figure 2.3 *The six dimensions of the Psychological General Well-being Index, presented with 95%-confidence intervals, as scored by migraine patients (n = 138; shaded boxes) and age- and gender-matched controls (n = 138; open boxes). Reproduced from reference 1.*

CHAPTER 3

EPIDEMIOLOGY

What is the prevalence of migraine?

Prevalence refers to the percentage of people in a given population with a certain condition. With regard to migraine, a review of studies conducted prior to the publication of the International Headache Society classification in 1988, revealed its prevalence to be 9% in men and 16% in women[2] (Figure 3.1). In children, the prevalence is 3-4% and is the same for boys as it is for girls. The review indicated the *incidence* of severe headache of migrainous and non-migrainous nature to be approximately 1%. This is the percentage of the population that becomes sufferers of severe headache on an annual basis.

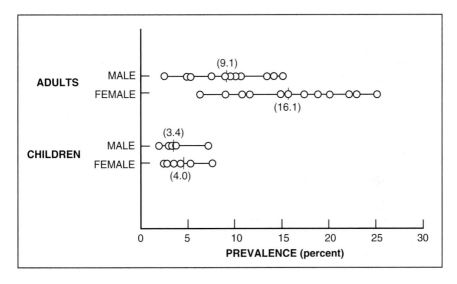

Figure 3.1. *Prevalence of migraine in the general population; the numbers in parentheses indicate the average values. Reproduced from reference 2.*

The review also showed the prevalence of migraine to sharply increase during the second decade of life[2]. It subsequently levels off and remains stable until the fourth or fifth decade, after which it slowly but steadily decreases (Figure 3.2). In women, the decrease in migraine prevalence

M‌IGRAINE

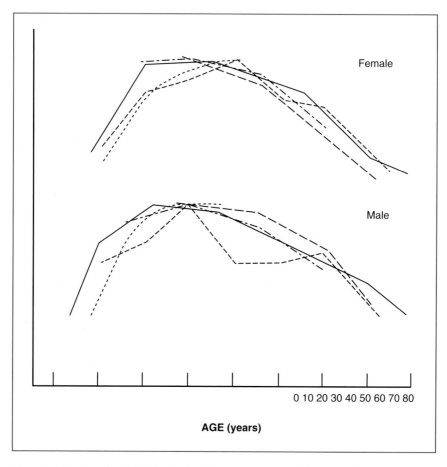

Figure 3.2. *Prevalence profile of migraine in relation to age, separately for men and women. Reproduced from reference 2.*

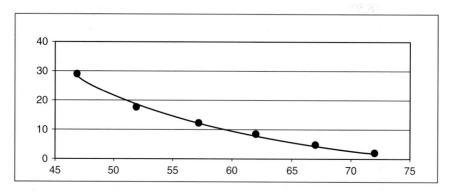

Figure 3.3. *Last-year prevalence of migraine, in percentage, in women aged 45 to 74 years. Data obtained from reference 5.*

after the age of 45 is exponential in nature[5] (Figure 3.3). The difference in prevalence between men and women reveals itself in the second decade of life, probably due to the onset of menstruation in women. In the review, the factors that were found to be significantly associated with headache, including migraine, were age, gender, stress, and anxiety/depression.

Application of the International Headache Society criteria to a random sample of the Danish population revealed the last-year prevalence of migraine to be 6% in men and 15% in women[6]. 'Last-year prevalence' refers to the occurrence of the condition in the preceding year. In the same study, it was found that the last-year prevalence of tension-type headache is 63% in men and 86% in women, chronic tension-type headache 3%, and cluster headache 0.14%. In the United States, application of simplified International Headache Society criteria and considering severe headaches only showed the last-year prevalence of migraine to be 6% in men and 18% in women[7]. The last-year prevalence of (self-defined) severe headache was 20%, affecting 13% of men and 26% of women. With a last-year prevalence of 12%, migraine accounted for a little over half of the severe headaches; one wonders to what the remaining severe headaches were due!

The study conducted in the United States revealed the last-year prevalence of migraine to be the highest in the age group of 35-45 years[7]. In addition, the study showed it to be inversely related to annual household income, which means that in the lowest income group (<$10,000/£6,100/€11,000), it was more than 60% higher than in the two highest income groups (>$30,000/£18,300/€33,000). The study did not reveal the last-year prevalence of migraine to be different between white and black race, urban and rural residence, and region of residence within the United States. The study was repeated 10 years later in 1999 with similar findings, that is, a last-year prevalence of severe headache of 21% and migraine of 13%[3].

The American Migraine Study II also provided information with regard to the basic variables, that is, frequency, intensity, and duration, of migraine headache in the general population[3]. With regard to frequency, it was found that the headaches occur less than once per month in 38%, between one and three times per month in 36%, and more than three times per month in 26%. The intensity of the headaches was mild in 2%, moderate in 34%, and severe in 64%. With regard to their duration, the migraine headaches were indicated to be shorter than 12 hours in 76%, between 12 and 24 hours in 12%, and longer than 24 hours in 12%. These findings suggest that in the general population, almost two-third of migraine sufferers experience headaches more than once per month. The headaches are generally severe in intensity but relatively short in duration, lasting less than 12 hours.

What is the current state of migraine treatment?

Many of those who have migraine unfortunately never seek medical consultation. This is unfortunate because migraine headaches typically do *not* respond to non-prescription medications, resulting in needless suffering. It is also regrettable from a public-health perspective because lack of effective abortive treatment over time increases the frequency of the headaches, potentially to daily occurrence. Daily headaches affect as much as 6% of the population and an estimated half of the daily headache sufferers initially experienced intermittent migraine headaches[8]. The progression is due to a gradual increase in tightness of the head and neck muscles, an inevitable consequence of the repeated occurrence of unmitigated migraine headaches.

Due to its hereditary nature, migraine is often present in the family and, therefore, familiar to the sufferer who knows that its prognosis is medically benign. With regard to the potential of obtaining relief, there is generally the implicit understanding that migraine cannot be cured. However, there often also seems to be the belief that the medical profession cannot do anything for the headaches that the sufferer cannot do him or herself. A population study conducted in the United States in 1989 underscored the extent to which migraine is both underdiagnosed and undertreated[4]. It showed that 71% of men and 59% of women identified with migraine in the general population did not have a physician diagnosis (Figure 3.4). This, despite the fact that all of them had severe headaches and, in addition, 80% experienced at least some degree of disability from them.

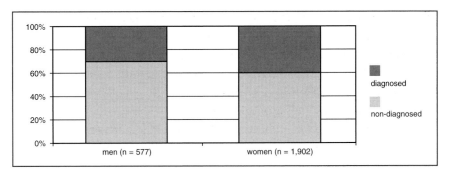

Figure 3.4. *Diagnosed versus non-diagnosed migraine in the general population, separately for men and women. Data obtained from reference 4.*

The symptoms most frequently associated with a physician diagnosis were vomiting, blurred vision, and a visual or sensory aura. A physician diagnosis was less likely if the annual household income was $10,000/£6,500/€11,000 or less. With regard to medication intake, the study revealed that most patients with migraine, 67% of men and 57% of women, rely on non-prescription medications to treat their headaches[1] (Figure 3.5). These numbers are very similar to the percentages of men and women in the general population with non-diagnosed migraine.

Only 28% of men and 40% of women took prescription medications and 5% of men and 3% of women took no medications at all. The highest use of prescription medications was found in those patients who experienced vomiting or a visual aura with their headaches, which were also the symptoms associated with physician diagnosis. The use of prescription medications was also related to the frequency and duration of the headaches, as well as to the extent of disability caused by them.

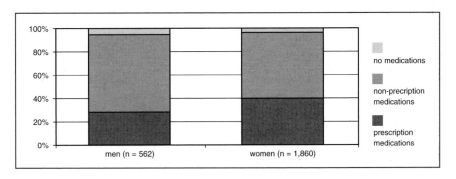

Figure 3.5. *Medication use for migraine in the general population, separately for men and women. Data obtained from reference 1.*

MIGRAINE

CHAPTER 4

CLASSIFICATION

How is migraine classified?

In the headache classification as proposed in 1962 by the National Institute of Neurological Diseases and Blindness, migraine is classified under "vascular headaches of the migraine type"[1]. This category includes classic migraine, common migraine, cluster headache, hemiplegic and ophthalmoplegic migraine, and lower-half headache (facial migraine). The headache conditions in this category are considered to have in common *extra*cranial arterial vasodilation as the mechanism causing the pain. The so-called Ad Hoc Committee classification was an attempt to classify headache on the basis of presumed underlying mechanisms. The following is the description of the vascular headaches of the migraine type, as it appears in the classification: *Recurrent attacks of headache widely varied in intensity, frequency, and duration. The attacks are commonly unilateral in onset; are usually associated with anorexia and, sometimes, with nausea and vomiting; in some are preceded by, or associated with, conspicuous sensory, motor, and mood disturbances; and are often familial.*

In the headache classification as proposed in 1988 by the International Headache Society, migraine represents a separate category with seven subcategories, as is shown in Table 4.1[2]. The two major subcategories are migraine *without* aura and migraine *with* aura, corresponding to common and classic migraine, respectively, of the Ad Hoc Committee classification. The International Headache Society classification does not concern itself with underlying mechanisms; it is purely descriptive and phenomenological and reduces headache diagnosis to a cookbook approach.

MIGRAINE

Table 4.1. *Subclassification of migraine by the International Headache Society2*

1.1	Migraine without aura
1.2	Migraine with aura
1.3	Ophthalmoplegic migraine
1.4	Retinal migraine
1.5	Childhood periodic syndromes
1.6	Complications of migraine
1.7	Migrainous disorders not fulfilling the above criteria

What are the diagnostic criteria for migraine without aura?

In its classification, the International Headache Society proposes strict criteria for the diagnosis of each of the headache conditions included. However, while strict criteria are important in research, they are *not* in patient care where the criteria should be used as guidelines only and clinical judgment should prevail. To arrive at the diagnosis of migraine without aura, the classification requires at least five headaches fulfilling the following criteria: *The headaches last for 4-72 hours although in children below the age of 15, they may be as short as two hours. They have to have at least two of the following four features: unilateral location, pulsating quality, moderate or severe intensity, and aggravation by walking stairs or similar routine physical activity.* (The intensity of the headaches is rated as moderate when they inhibit and severe when they prohibit daily activities.) *The headaches are associated with nausea or vomiting or with photophobia and phonophobia.* The criteria are listed in Table 4.2.

Table 4.2. *Diagnostic criteria for migraine without aura as proposed by the International Headache Society*[2]

A.   At least five headaches fulfilling conditions B-D

B.   The headaches last for 4-72 hours (untreated or unsuccessfully treated)

C.   The headaches have at least two of the following features:

    1.   Unilateral location

    2.   Pulsating quality

    3.   Moderate or severe intensity

    4.   Aggravation by walking stairs or similar routine physical activity

D.   During the headaches, at least one of the following is present:

    1. Nausea or vomiting

    2. Photophobia and phonophobia

Case studies of migraine without aura

A 32-year-old woman has experienced headaches since her teens. The headaches occur three or four times per month. They are present on awakening in the morning or come on during the day. The headaches build to their maximum intensity in two to three hours and last for 12 hours. They are located in the forehead, eye, and temple, on the left or on the right, without preference. The headaches are moderate or severe in intensity and associated with photophobia and phonophobia. Once or twice per year, they are also associated with nausea and vomiting. Light and noise make the headaches worse and lying down in a cool, dark, and quiet room makes them somewhat better.

A 35-year-old woman has experienced headaches since age 21, when she started taking an oral contraceptive. The headaches occur once per month during the withdrawal bleeding. They come on during the day, build to their maximum intensity in one day, and last for three to four days.

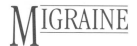

The headaches are located on the left and extend from the back of the head into the eye. They are severe in intensity and sharp, steady in nature. The headaches are associated with nausea, vomiting, photophobia, and phonophobia. Lying down in a dark room and applying ice to the head make them somewhat better.

What are the diagnostic criteria for migraine with aura?

The diagnosis of migraine with aura is based on the aura and not on the headache; hence, the features of the headaches are irrelevant (*sic!*). The classification of the International Headache Society requires at least two attacks, which fulfill three of the following four criteria: *There are one or more fully reversible aura symptoms indicating focal cerebrocortical or brainstem dysfunction. At least one aura symptom develops gradually over more than 4 minutes or two or more symptoms occur in succession. No aura symptom lasts longer than 60 minutes but if more than one aura symptom is present, the accepted duration is proportionally increased. The headache follows the aura with a symptom-free interval of less than 60 minutes but may also begin before or simultaneously with the aura.* The criteria are listed in Table 4.3.

Table 4.3. *Diagnostic criteria for migraine with aura as proposed by the International Headache Society[2]*

A. At least two attacks fulfilling B
B. At least three of the following four characteristics are present:
1. One or more fully reversible aura symptoms indicating focal cerebrocortical or brainstem dysfunction
2. At least one aura symptom develops gradually over more than 4 minutes or two or more symptoms occur in succession
3. No aura symptom lasts longer than 60 minutes but if more than one aura symptom is present, the accepted duration is proportionally increased
4. The headache follows the aura with a symptom-free interval of less than 60 minutes but may also begin before or simultaneously with the aura

Case studies of migraine with aura

A 27-year-old woman has experienced headaches since age 13, when she started menstruating. The headaches occur once per month perimenstrually and sometimes also with ovulation. They come on during the day, build to their maximum intensity in one half to one hour, and last for one to two days. The headaches are severe in intensity and associated with nausea, irritability, photophobia, phonophobia, and osmophobia. They are located in the right eye, temple, and back of the head. The headaches begin as a sharp, steady pain, which gradually becomes dull and throbbing. They are preceded by a visual disturbance, which lasts for 15-20 minutes. The disturbance affects both visual fields but is more pronounced on the left. It consists of diagonal zigzag lines, which move across both visual fields from the bottom right to the top left. The zigzag lines are white-silver; they flicker and look like lightning.

A 55-year-old man has experienced headaches since age 14. The headaches occur once per week and last for one to two days. They come on in the course of the morning and build to their maximum intensity in 30 minutes. The headaches begin in the frontotemporal area on one side or the other and from there become generalized. They are usually moderate in intensity and associated with nausea, photophobia, phonophobia, and blurred vision. The headaches are preceded by a visual disturbance, consisting of distortion of vision, bright lights, and lightning patterns. The visual disturbance begins in one visual field or the other but always on the side, opposite to the ensuing headache. After its onset and like the headache, the visual disturbance becomes generalized to involve both visual fields. It lasts for half an hour and is immediately followed by headache.

What is the significance of the migraine with aura subcategories?

In general practice, the subcategories of migraine with aura as distinguished by the International Headache Society and shown in Table 4.4 are probably of little significance. An exception is the subcategory referred to as *migraine aura without headache* (1.2.5), in which the aura symptoms are not followed by headache. This is a relatively common condition, which, especially in the older patient, needs to be differentiated from *transient ischemic attacks*.

MIGRAINE

Table 4.4. *Subcategories of migraine with aura as proposed by the International Headache Society*[2]

1.2.1	Migraine with typical aura
1.2.2	Migraine with prolonged aura
1.2.3	Familial hemiplegic migraine
1.2.4	Basilar migraine
1.2.5	Migraine aura without headache
1.2.6	Migraine with acute onset aura

In migraine with prolonged aura (1.2.2), one or more of the aura symptoms last longer than 60 minutes but shorter than one week and neuroimaging is normal. If neuroimaging is abnormal, that is, shows ischemic infarction, or one or more of the aura symptoms last longer than one week, migrainous infarction is diagnosed (1.6.2). Migrainous infarction is a subcategory of complications of migraine (1.6) (Table 4.1) but can also occur in migraine without aura, although this is not recognized in the classification[4]. However, migraine aura symptoms can last longer than one week *without* being associated with cerebral infarction. This is referred to as *migraine aura status*, a condition also not included in the classification[5]!

Case studies of migraine with prolonged aura

A 22-year-old woman has experienced headaches since age 12. The headaches occur once per two to three months and last for 24-72 hours. They begin as a pressure across the forehead, within 10-15 minutes followed by a visual disturbance, which lasts for two to four hours. The visual disturbance affects both visual fields and consists of white and blue, flickering zigzag lines and white flickering dots. As soon as the visual disturbance begins, the pain localizes to one side or the other. The headaches are throbbing in nature and builds to their maximum intensity in several minutes. They are associated with nausea, photophobia, and phonophobia.

A 27-year-old man has experienced headaches since age 13. The headaches occur five to six times during two week episodes with remissions of one to two months. They build to their maximum intensity in 20-30 minutes and last for two to three hours. The headaches are located in the sides of the head and are sharp, steady in nature. They are moderate in intensity and associated with photophobia. The headaches are preceded by a visual disturbance, which consists of bright, diagonal lines in one visual field or the other. The visual disturbance begins as an after-image of a bright light and develops over 10-15 minutes. It lasts for 20 minutes and gradually fades away after it is fully developed. In 90% the visual disturbance is followed by headache, which comes on 15-20 minutes later. The headache always occurs contralateral to the visual disturbance. On one occasion, the visual disturbance occurred twice in the course of one hour. The second time, the diagonal lines occurred in both visual fields and lasted for three to four hours. After the diagonal lines cleared, the periphery of both visual fields remained blurred for two days.

Migraine aura status refers to aura symptoms that last longer than one week but are not associated with cerebral infarction. As mentioned before, it is a migraine condition that is not included in the International Headache Society classification.

Case study of migraine aura status

A 41-year-old man has experienced headaches since childhood. The headaches occur twelve to fifteen times per year, often in episodes. They are always preceded by a visual disturbance, which lasts for 20-40 minutes. The visual disturbance consists of bright-white, flickering zigzag lines ("white snakes") in the periphery of both visual fields. It develops over 5-10 minutes and is immediately followed by headache. The headache builds to its maximum intensity as the visual disturbance fades away and lasts for half to one hour, treated with a non-prescription analgesic. The headache is severe in intensity, located in the anterior vertex as a throbbing pain, and is associated with photophobia. In October 1996, he was watching Clinton's re-election on television, which upset him greatly. He subsequently developed the visual disturbance as described above but much more intense. It was associated with tingling of his left arm and hand, which developed without a march and lasted for 15-30 minutes. It was associated with severe headache, photophobia, and a general sense of weakness. In addition, he was confused and kept repeating the same sentence. The visual disturbance has been present ever since, affecting his vision as if he is looking through a veil. The "white snakes" in the periphery of both visual fields come and go. Cranial magnetic-resonance imaging was normal and without evidence of infarction.

In migraine with acute onset aura (1.2.6), the aura symptoms develop fully within 4 minutes. However, the acute onset of the aura symptoms may be more the result of inaccurate history taking than reflecting their true development.

Familial hemiplegic migraine (1.2.3) is a rare (childhood) condition of recurrent headaches associated with hemiparesis. An additional prerequisite for the diagnosis is that at least one first-degree relative is affected as well. It also occurs in a non-familial form, which, again, the International Headache Society does not recognize in its classification. It is important that the hemiparesis is *not* associated with paresthesias. Otherwise, the weakness can be due solely to the somatosensory disturbance and does not necessarily imply motor involvement.

Case study of (non-familial) hemiplegic migraine

A 37-year-old woman has experienced headaches since age 10. The headaches occur two or three times per month and last for two to three days. They are present on awakening in the morning or come on during the day. The headaches build to their maximum intensity in one hour. They are severe in intensity and sharp, steady in nature. The headaches are located on one side or the other, with a preference for the right. They often begin in the side of the nose and extend from there to behind the eye. Sometimes the headaches begin in the back of the neck. They are associated with photophobia and phonophobia, as well as with throbbing in the temple on the side of the pain. When the headaches start during the day, a feeling of weakness in the ipsilateral arm and hand precedes them. The weakness is not associated with loss of feeling, numbness, or tingling. It begins one hour before the onset of the headaches and lasts for their full duration.

Basilar (artery) migraine (1.2.4) is, like hemiplegic migraine, a rare condition that mostly affects young adults. In basilar migraine, the aura symptoms originate from the brainstem and are often alarming in nature, such as double vision, bilateral numbness or tingling, or drowsiness. The condition needs to be differentiated from migraine associated with hyperventilation or vasovagal lability. Symptoms of hyperventilation are lightheadedness and a feeling of numbness or tingling in both hands and around the mouth; those of vasovagal lability are lightheadedness and seeing black before the eyes.

Case study of basilar (artery) migraine

A 22-year-old man has experienced headaches since age nine. The headaches occur once per month and last for 24-72 hours. They come on during the day and build to their maximum intensity in one to two hours. The headaches are located bilaterally in the temples and in the sides of the head, usually worse on the right. They are severe in intensity and sharp, pounding in the temples. The headaches are associated with nausea, photophobia, phonophobia, blurred vision, and vomiting to the point of dehydration. They are also associated with lightheadedness, confusion, irritability, slurred speech, double vision, and impaired coordination. The latter symptoms begin two to four hours before the onset of the headaches and last for their full duration.

What is retinal and ophthalmoplegic migraine?

Retinal migraine (1.4) is a form of migraine with aura although the International Headache Society classifies it as a separate condition. The aura symptoms are visual in nature but monocular, affecting an eye, rather than homonymous, affecting a visual field. They are also fully reversible, last shorter than 60 minutes, and are followed by headache after a symptom-free interval of less than 60 minutes. In ophthalmoplegic migraine (1.3), the headaches are associated with weakness of one or more of the extraocular muscles, resulting in double vision. The weakness is due to ocular nerve dysfunction, usually involving the oculomotor nerve but sometimes only its parasympathetic fibers, resulting in a dilated pupil unresponsive to light.

What is status migrainosus?

According to the International Headache Society classification, there are two complications of migraine: status migrainosus (1.6.1), or migraine status, and migrainous infarction (1.6.2), also referred to as complicated migraine. Status migrainosus is the term used when a migraine headache lasts longer than 72 hours, although a headache-free interval of less than four hours may occur between consecutive headaches.

Case study of status migrainosus

A 51-year-old woman has experienced headaches since age 36, following a pregnancy. Initially, the headaches occurred once per month with menstruation and lasted for 24-48 hours. They were severe in intensity but not associated with nausea or vomiting. When she started taking an oral contraceptive, the headaches became longer lasting. They occurred during the placebo week and lasted for five to seven days. Since discontinuing the oral contraceptive two to three months ago, she has had a severe headache daily. The headache is located in the left forehead, eye, and side of the nose and is sharp, steady in nature. It is associated with photophobia, mostly in the left eye, and phonophobia. The headache is made worse by physical activity, bending over, and watching television. Lying down quietly in a dark room and applying ice to the left side of the face make it somewhat better.

A migraine status can often be effectively treated with a short course of a corticosteroid. I prefer prednisone, which I prescribe in a three-day course: 15 mg four times per day for one day, 10 mg four times per day for one day, and 5 mg four times per day for one day. It is important that as soon as the corticosteroid treatment is started, *all* abortive medications are discontinued. Full relief of headache usually occurs within 24 hours of initiation of the treatment. Possible side effects of corticosteroids are heartburn, stomach pain, nervousness, and insomnia; contraindications are active infection and recent vaccination.

What is complicated migraine?

Complicated migraine is a migraine attack complicated by ischemic stroke, which, according to the International Headache Society classification, can only occur in migraine with aura. This is not correct, however, because the complication of migraine by stroke is independent of the occurrence of aura symptoms. It is, in fact, more related to the intensity of the headache and its associated symptoms, nausea and vomiting, resulting in dehydration, than to the occurrence of aura. The pathogenesis of stroke in migraine is also different from that of the aura symptoms: while the aura symptoms are caused by a primary neuronal disturbance, the stroke is the result of cerebral vasospasm.

Case study of complicated migraine

A 30-year-old woman has experienced headaches since age 16, when she hit a tree riding her motor bike. The headaches occur seven or eight times per year and usually come on in the late afternoon. They gradually build in intensity to reach their maximum in the early evening, forcing her to retire early. The headaches are located in the right temple and are throbbing in nature. They are not associated with nausea, vomiting, photophobia, or phonophobia. One early evening, she retired with a headache but became nauseated and vomited all night. She also noticed tingling in the left side of her body. The following morning she had difficulty seeing off to the left with either eye. The headache and tingling persisted for the entire day. On examination, she had a left homonymous hemianopia with sparing of central vision. Cranial computerized tomography without contrast revealed an infarct in the territory of the right calcarine artery. Angiography showed irregular narrowing of the right posterior cerebral artery, suggestive of vasospasm (Figure 4.1).

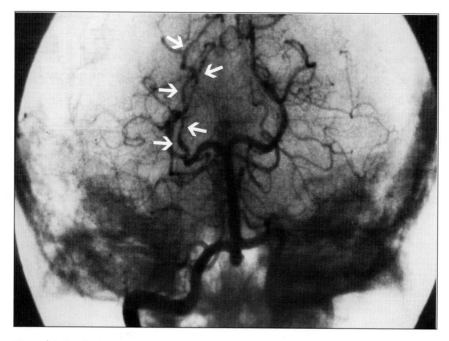

Figure 4.1. *Vertebral angiogram, showing vasospasm (arrows) of the right posterior cerebral artery in a patient with migraine (without aura) complicated by stroke. Reproduced from reference 5.*

CHAPTER 5

SYMPTOMATOLOGY

What are the symptoms of migraine?

The symptoms of migraine are limited to the migraine attack; in between the attacks, the patient is symptom-free. The central symptom of the migraine attack is headache, although it is sometimes absent as in migraine aura without headache. The headache of migraine is generally so intense that it interferes with the ability to function or may be incapacitating and require bed rest. In most cases, it is limited to one side of the head and alternates sides, although it may have a preference for one side or the other. It is often located in the temple and may also occur sometimes in or behind the eye (Figure 5.1). Other preferential locations of the migraine headache are in the forehead and in the back of the head, often just behind the ear.

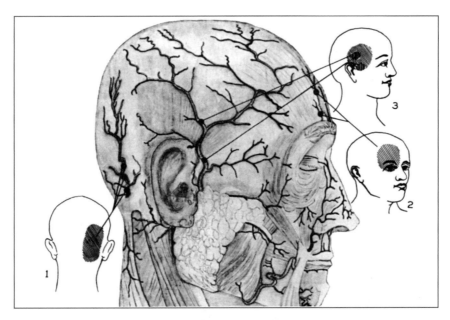

Figure 5.1. *Preferential locations of the migraine headache in relation to the extracranial arteries, that is, the occipital (1), supraorbital (2), and (superficial) temporal artery (3). Reproduced from reference 1.*

MIGRAINE

The headache of migraine is throbbing or sharp steady in nature, especially in the temple. Motion and activity aggravate it and may bring out the throbbing quality of the pain; the same can happen with bending over, coughing, sneezing, or straining. The headache is generally made somewhat better by lying down, although not entirely flat, and by applying pressure or cold to the temple, eye, or forehead.

What are the symptoms associated with the migraine headache?

The migraine headache is almost always associated with other symptoms. These symptoms occur after the onset of the headache and generally build in intensity as the headache progresses. The associated symptoms can be divided into autonomic and sensory. The autonomic symptoms consist of paleness of the face, coldness of the hands and feet, lack of appetite, nausea, vomiting, and diarrhea. They are due to activation of the sympathetic nervous system caused by the pain[2]. The sensory symptoms consist of photophobia, phonophobia, and osmophobia. The increased sensitivity to light and noise can be so intense that exposure to them increases the intensity of the pain. The increased sensitivity to smell, even when pleasant, for example perfume, can aggravate the nausea and cause vomiting.

The exact cause of the sensory symptoms is not known but they are probably also secondary to the headache. They may be due to the increased arousal caused by the pain through stimulation of the ascending reticular activating system. However, a peripheral mechanism may also be involved in the photophobia, consisting of relaxation of the muscles of accommodation. These muscles have a rudimentary sympathetic innervation, which is activated, as mentioned above, secondary to the pain. The involvement of this particular mechanism may also explain the blurred vision, especially near vision, which can be seen during migraine headache[3]. It is often not recognized as an associated symptom of the headache and is regularly mistaken for an aura symptom.

What are the aura symptoms of migraine?

In migraine with aura, the headache is preceded by transient focal neurological symptoms, called aura symptoms. They are almost always sensory in nature and occur before the onset of the headache or during the initial phase of headache development. They are relatively short in duration and generally last for 20 minutes, with a range of 10-30 minutes.

The aura symptoms of migraine are most often visual in nature but can also be somatosensory. A typical presentation of the visual aura of migraine is the scintillating scotoma, also referred to as fortification spectra or teichopsia (Figure 5.2; above). It usually begins near the center of vision as a twinkling star, which develops into a circle of bright and sometimes colorful flickering zigzag lines. The circle opens up on the inside to form a semicircle or horseshoe, which further expands into the periphery of one visual field or the other. On the inside of the visual disturbance, a band of dimness follows in the wake of the crescent of flickering zigzag lines. The disturbance of vision ultimately disappears as it fades away, or moves outside, the visual field in which it developed.

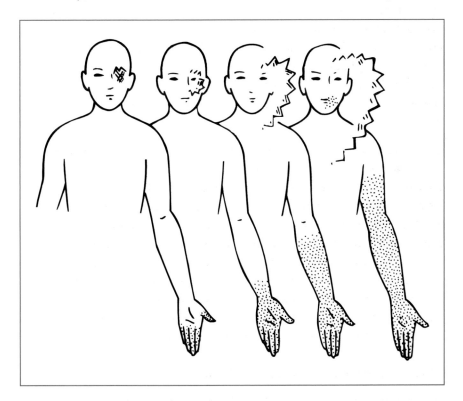

Figure 5.2. *Scintillating scotoma (above) and digitolingual paresthesias (below), shown from left to right in their successive stages of development.*

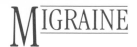

MIGRAINE

What is the presentation of the somatosensory disturbance?

The typical presentation of the somatosensory disturbance of migraine consists of digitolingual or cheiro-oral paresthesias (Figure 5.2; below), a sensation of numbness or tingling. It typically starts in the fingers of one hand, extending upward into the arm and, at a certain point, also involving the nose-mouth area on the same side. The progression of the somatosensory disturbance, like that of the scintillating scotoma, is slow and usually takes 10-30 minutes. A similarly progressing somatosensory disturbance can occur with stroke, although this is rare. What differentiates one from the other is the resolution of the disturbed sensation, to which the first-last rule applies: in migraine, what is involved first, resolves first while in stroke, what is involved first resolves last. This particular difference relates to the different mechanisms involved, which is spreading cortical excitation/depression in migraine and ischemic corticoneuronal dysfunction in stroke.

The digitolingual paresthesias are *always* unilateral and should be differentiated from the bilateral tingling in the hands and around the mouth, typical for hyperventilation syndrome. The tingling is sometimes so intense that the involved extremity is perceived as weak but examination will disprove this. If real muscle weakness exists and sensation is intact, the condition is either that of hemiplegic migraine or migrainous infarction. Both migraine conditions are rare and hemiplegic migraine mostly occurs in childhood. Migrainous infarction is a migraine attack complicated by stroke and is also referred to as complicated migraine. It is a one-time event that needs to be treated as a stroke with symptomatic treatment of the headache only. When occurring during a migraine attack, the stroke usually results in homonymous hemianopia rather than in hemiparesis, as is generally the case with stroke. Unfortunately, it often leaves the patient with a permanent neurological deficit, although usually improvement occurs over time due to the relatively young age at which stroke occurs in migraine.

Case study of migraine with aura

A 17-year-old woman has experienced headaches since age six to seven. Generally, the headaches occur once per two weeks although sometimes three or four times per week. They come on during the day and last for five to six hours. The headaches are located in the temple and behind the eye, on one side or the other without preference. They are severe in intensity and throbbing in nature. The headaches are associated with pallor, nausea, vomiting, photophobia, phonophobia, and frequent urination. They are preceded by a visual disturbance, which lasts for 30 minutes. The visual disturbance sometimes consists of an obscuration, like a mist, of one visual field or the other. At other times, it begins as an obscuration of central vision, surrounded by a circle of bright and flickering zigzag lines. As it expands, the circle of zigzag lines brakes up into segments, which move toward the periphery of both visual fields. In the periphery of the visual fields, the segments of zigzag lines transform into vertical wavy lines, which gradually fade away. The attacks are precipitated by bright, especially fluorescent light, watching television, stress, and heat.

A 35-year-old woman has experienced headaches since age nine. The headaches occur once every three weeks. They are preceded by a visual disturbance, consisting of an area of grayness in the center of vision. On the right of the grayness, a crescent of flickering zigzag lines develops, which gradually expands toward the periphery of the right visual field. As the crescent moves across the visual field, the grayness moves along with it as a band lying against the inside. The visual disturbance lasts for one hour and is immediately followed by headache. The headaches are usually located in the right temple but are sometimes located on the left. They are severe in intensity, steady in nature, and associated with nausea and occasionally also with vomiting. The headaches last for 36 hours and are precipitated by going without food too long, strong odors, and exercise. When she was taking an oral contraceptive, the visual disturbance was associated with a feeling of tingling. The tingling started in the left hand and gradually extended upward into the forearm, ultimately skipping to the left side of the face, especially affecting the nose, mouth, tongue, and palate. On one occasion, she also experienced slurred speech and difficulty forming words along with the visual disturbance.

A 37-year-old man has experienced headaches since age nine. The headaches occur every three weeks. They build to their maximum intensity in one hour and last for one to three days. The headaches are severe in intensity and located bilaterally in the temples. They are associated with pallor but not with nausea, vomiting, photophobia, or phonophobia. The headaches are made somewhat better by lying down quietly and are made worse by suddenly moving the head. They are always preceded by a feeling of tingling, which starts in the fingers of one hand. The tingling extends upward and in 10 minutes involves the entire arm. It is so pronounced that it becomes difficult for him to use his arm and hand. When affecting the left, the tingling moves downward from the shoulder into the chest and leg. The progression of the sensory disturbance from the left hand to the left foot takes 30 minutes.

What is abdominal migraine?

Abdominal migraine is a chronic condition of recurring abdominal symptoms, including nausea, vomiting, diarrhea, and abdominal pain. It has been linked to migraine because of its functional nature, its simultaneous occurrence with migraine, or migraine occurring in the family. Sometimes, it precedes the onset of migraine and, therefore, is also considered a migraine forerunner. The diagnosis should be made by the exclusion of numerous other causes of recurring abdominal symptoms, ranging from constipation to inborn errors of metabolism. It should also be differentiated from chronic non-recurring abdominal symptoms, occurring due to a variety of causes as well, including chronic rhinosinusitis!

Children who suffer from migraine tend to have more associated abdominal symtoms with their attacks.

Case study of abdominal migraine

A 37-year-old woman has experienced headaches since age 18. The headaches occur once every 3-12 months and last for 8-10 hours. They come on mid-morning and build to their maximum intensity in half an hour. The headaches are severe in intensity and associated with severe nausea, photophobia, and occasionally also with vomiting. They are located behind the right eye as a sharp, steady pain. Movement and activity make the nausea worse and lying down makes it somewhat better and prevents vomiting. Lack of sleep and not eating on time bring on headache. The headaches are preceded by a visual disturbance, which lasts for half an hour and consists of loss of vision in the right, upper visual field. Since her late twenties, she has also experienced attacks of nausea without headache and without visual disturbance. These attacks occur once per month and are also brought on by lack of sleep and not eating on time. Like the headaches, they start mid-morning and last until early evening. The nausea is so intense that it forces her to lie down; vomiting temporarily relieves it. The headaches as well as the nausea attacks responded preventively to treatment with amitriptyline, 50 mg at bedtime.

What is exertional migraine?

Exertional migraine is a condition in which migraine headaches are (almost) exclusively brought on by physical exertion. It is seen especially in children with the addition of other trigger factors, in particular fatigue, as the child grows older. Exertion as a trigger of migraine headache probably results from overheating of the body, causing extracranial vasodilation, and tends to be more common with hot and humid weather. Treatment is often effective with a non-steroidal anti-inflammatory analgesic, such as ibuprofen, 400 mg, or naproxen sodium, 440 mg, taken half to one hour before the physical activity. In adults, a similar condition is seen with sexual activity, whether intercourse or masturbation. The headache occurs more or less abruptly during orgasm as a result of the increase in blood pressure, causing the extracranial vasodilation. It should be distinguished from the headache that develops gradually during sexual activity as a result of increasing muscle tightness, due to sustained extension of the neck.

Case study of exertional migraine

A 12-year-old boy has experienced headaches since age seven. The headaches occur whenever he exerts himself physically for more than 30 minutes, for example, playing tennis, soccer, or baseball, especially when the weather is hot and humid. They come on during the exercise, build to their maximum intensity in five minutes after he stops exercising, and last for the remainder of the day. The headaches are located in the forehead and anterior vertex and are like a steady pressure during the exertion but throbbing afterwards. Prior to the onset of headache during exertion, he feels tired and hot and his face looks red. In 20%, the headaches are associated with nausea, vomiting, phonophobia, and sometimes also with bright spots in front of the eyes. Bending over and caffeine make them worse while taking a cold shower and sleeping make them better. His mother has been diagnosed with migraine; his father and sister also have headaches.

CHAPTER 6

PATHOGENESIS

What is the pathogenesis of the migraine headache?

There is *clinical* experimental evidence that at least three mechanisms are involved in the pathogenesis of the migraine headache. These mechanisms are *extra*cranial arterial vasodilation, *extra*cranial neurogenic inflammation, and decreased inhibition of central pain transmission.

In the 1930s, Graham and Wolff were the first to study the mechanism of extracranial arterial vasodilation in the pathogenesis of the migraine headache[6]. They observed that pressure exerted on the extracranial arteries temporarily decreases the intensity of the pain. In addition, they found that administration of ergotamine results in a decrease in intensity of the headache, parallel to a decrease in pulsation amplitude of the *extra*cranial arteries. It was also observed that increasing the pressure of the cerebrospinal fluid by intrathecal injection of saline, thereby decreasing the pulsation amplitude of the intracranial arteries, does *not* decrease the intensity of the pain[16]. This suggests that the intracranial arteries, cerebral or extracerebral, that is, dural or meningeal, do not significantly contribute to the pain of the migraine headache.

The artery that seems to be predominantly involved in the mechanism of migrainous vasodilation is the frontal branch of the superficial temporal artery, giving rise to the pain in the temple so characteristic of migraine. In 1953, Tunis and Wolff reported on the systolic pulse-wave amplitude of the frontal branch of the superficial temporal artery in migraineurs during and between headaches and in non-headache controls[19] (Figure 6.1). They found the amplitude, taken as a measure of artery caliber, to be significantly increased in between headaches in comparison to controls, with a further increase during headache.

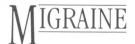

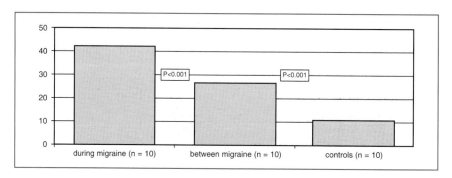

Figure 6.1. *Systolic pulse-wave amplitude of the frontal branch of the superficial temporal artery, in mm (amplified), during and between migraine headaches and in non-headache controls. Data obtained from reference 19.*

More recent clinical experimental evidence for the involvement of the temporal artery in the pathogenesis of the migraine headache is shown in Figure 6.2[8]. It shows that during the migraine headache, the artery is dilated on the side of the pain in comparison to the other side. The dilation is relative because generalized vasoconstriction occurs due to the activation of the sympathetic nervous system, secondary to the pain of the migraine headache. The generalized vasoconstriction causes the paleness of the face and coldness of the hands and feet, often seen during migraine headache. The fact that patients with migraine have dilated temporal arteries also in between headaches was recently confirmed as well, as is shown in Figure 6.3[4].

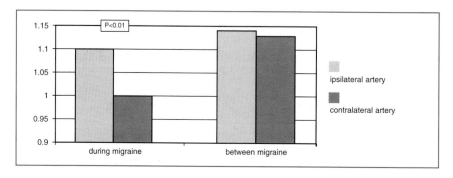

Figure 6.2. *Luminal diameter of the superficial temporal artery, in mm, during and between migraine, ipsilateral and contralateral to the headache (n = 25). Data obtained from reference 8.*

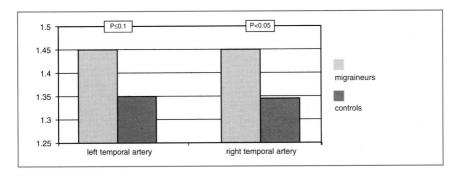

Figure 6.3. *Luminal diameter of the superficial temporal artery, in mm, in migraineurs between headaches (n = 50), in comparison to non-headache controls (n = 50). Data obtained from reference 4.*

What is neurogenic inflammation?

Neurogenic inflammation is inflammation of peripheral tissue, caused by the release of chemicals in the tissue from the primary sensory nerve fibers involved in pain transmission. The chemicals, which include substance P, calcitonin gene-related peptide, and neurokinin A, are released from the nerve fibers when they are activated. In migraine, the nerve-fiber activation results from the dilation of the extracranial arteries. The nerve fibers coil around the arteries and are stretched, thereby depolarized and activated, when the blood vessels dilate.

In the 1950s, Chapman and Wolff were the first to study neurogenic inflammation as a mechanism involved in the pathogenesis of the migraine headache[3]. They observed that subcutaneous perfusates of sites of migraine headache have inflammatory activity, proportional to the intensity of the pain (Figure 6.4). In addition, they found that administration of ergotamine results in a decrease in inflammatory activity, parallel to a decrease in intensity of the pain. More recently, it was shown that during migraine headache, the level of calcitonin gene-related peptide in the external jugular vein is increased, in comparison to the antecubital vein[5] (Figure 6.5). Calcitonin gene-related peptide is one of the chemicals involved in neurogenic inflammation; the external jugular vein drains blood from the extracranial tissues.

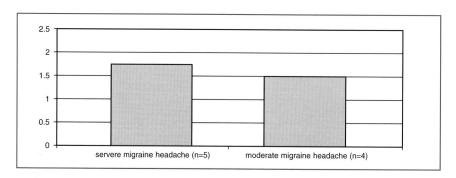

Figure 6.4. *Inflammatory activity of subcutaneous perfusates of sites of migraine headache, in bradykinin units, in relation to the intensity of the pain. Data obtained from reference 3.*

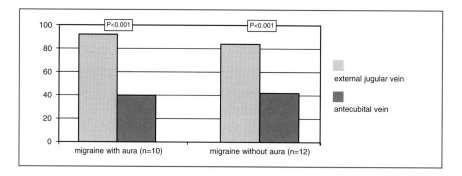

Figure 6.5. *Level of calcitonin gene-related peptide in blood drawn from the external jugular vein, in pmol/l, during migraine headaches in comparison to blood drawn from the antecubital vein. Data obtained from reference 5.*

The neurogenic inflammation results in a decrease in pain threshold at the site of the pain. This was first shown by Wolff *et al.* in 1953[22] (Figure 6.6) and has recently been confirmed as cutaneous allodynia occurring during migraine headache[2]. Allodynia refers to pain resulting from non-noxious stimulation of normal (looking) tissue and was found in the ipsilateral periorbital area during migraine headache in 79% of 42 patients studied.

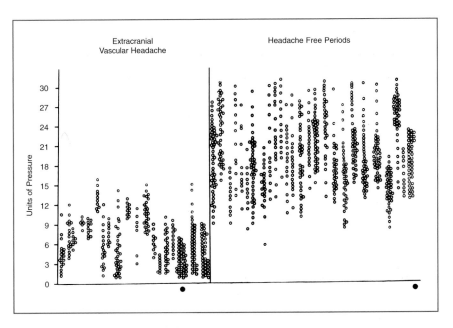

Figure 6.6. *Deep pain threshold measured in the area of pain during (left) and between migraine headaches (right)(n = 10). Reproduced from reference 22.*

Apart from neurogenic inflammation, there is probably also a central mechanism involved in the decrease in pain threshold at the site of the migraine headache. Evidence for this was provided by a study of the enkephalin level, determined in cerebrospinal fluid during migraine headache[1]. Enkephalin is an endogenous opioid and inhibits the transmission of pain signals in the central nervous system. It is decreased during migraine headache in comparison to between headaches and non-headache controls (Figure 6.7).

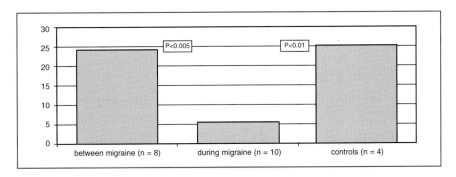

Figure 6.7. *Enkephalin level of the cerebrospinal fluid, in pmol equivalents of met-enkephalin/ml, during and between migraine headaches and in non-headache controls. Data obtained from reference 1.*

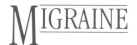

What is the pathogenesis of the migraine aura?

In the 1940s and 50s, Schumacher, Marcussen, and Wolff, were the first to experimentally study the pathogenesis of the migraine aura[9, 16]. They observed that inhalation of a cerebral vasodilator, such as amyl nitrite or carbon dioxide, during the migraine aura results in a transient regression of the symptoms (Figure 6.8). Hence, they concluded that the migraine aura is caused by transient cerebral vasoconstriction.

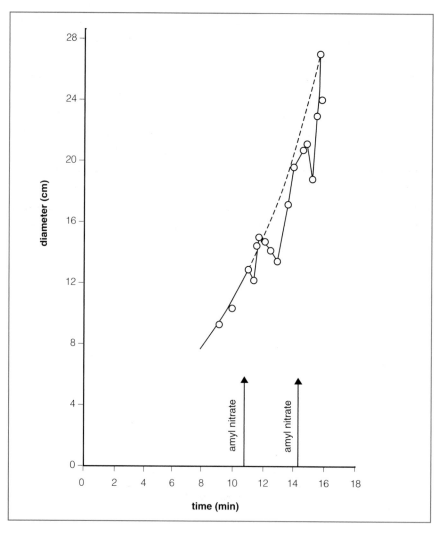

Figure 6.8. *Effect of the cerebral vasodilator, amyl nitrite, on the progression of the scintillating scotoma. Reproduced from reference 7.*

In 1958, Milner reported on the similarities in features and progression between the scintillating scotoma and spreading depression, a neurophysiological phenomenon described by Leão in 1944[10]. Spreading depression is a wave of inhibition of neuronal activity, which travels over the cerebral cortex at a slow rate. It is preceded by a short-lasting phase of intense neuronal activity and, therefore, is better referred to as "spreading excitation".

In the 1970s, relatively accurate measurement of cerebral blood flow became possible with the development of the Xenon-clearance technique. Olesen *et al* summarized the results of blood flow studies applying this technique, in 63 patients with attacks of migraine with aura triggered by angiography[11]. They concluded that the aura symptoms come on *after* a decrease in blood flow occurs in the posterior region of the opposite hemisphere. The headache comes on *while* blood flow is still decreased but is followed by a gradual increase in blood flow to an abnormally high level (Figure 6.9). The increase in cerebral blood flow that follows the decrease was initially attributed to reactive hyperemia. However, the decrease did *not* reach ischemic levels, required to cause reactive hyperemia, and was, therefore, referred to as oligemia[12]. The oligemia was shown to spread over the cerebral cortex at a slow rate, similar to Leão's spreading excitation/depression.

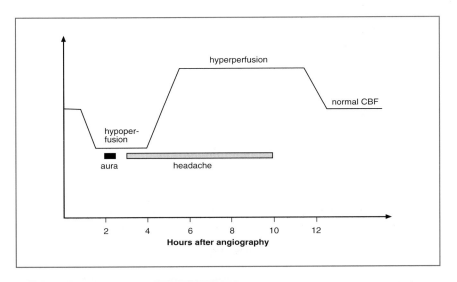

Figure 6.9. *Changes in cerebral blood flow in relation to the occurrence of the aura and headache in migraine with aura. Reproduced from reference 11.*

The development of functional magnetic-resonance imaging made it possible to study the changes in cerebral blood flow during spontaneous migraine attacks. The resolution of this method is also much better than that of the Xenon-clearance technique and, in addition, the brain can be studied in different planes. It was found that during the migraine aura, cerebral blood flow is decreased by 27% in the contralateral occipital cortex and this decrease persists for up to two and a half hours into the headache[15]. Whether cerebral blood flow subsequently increases, as suggested by the Xenon-clearance studies, is not clear. An increase of 20% over multiple attacks was observed in one of three patients studied. In the patients with migraine without aura, no changes in cerebral blood flow were found 1-11 hours after the onset of headache, as compared to in between headaches.

On the basis of the clinical presentation of the migraine aura, the mechanism involved is more likely to be spreading cortical excitation/depression, rather than transient cerebral vasoconstriction. This notion is supported by the results of brain spectroscopy, which showed an alteration in energy metabolism during migraine with aura but without changes in pH[21]. Cerebral vasoconstriction is the mechanism involved in migrainous infarction, which can complicate a migraine headache with or without aura[18].

What is the relationship between the aura and headache?

It is important to remember that only in the minority of cases, the migraine headache is preceded by an aura. Otherwise, we are dealing with migraine without aura, in which the headache occurs without aura but is otherwise the same. In the traditional view, the pathogenesis of the migraine aura and headache are considered causally related, that is, the aura is considered to be the *cause* of the headache. The aura is related to cerebral vasoconstriction, which causes localized hypoxia of the brain and is followed by reactive vasodilation. The vasodilation occurs in the cerebral circulation but is supposedly associated with dilation of extracranial arteries. The extracranial arterial vasodilation initiates the mechanism of neurogenic inflammation and the interplay of the two generates the pain of the migraine headache (Figure 6.10).

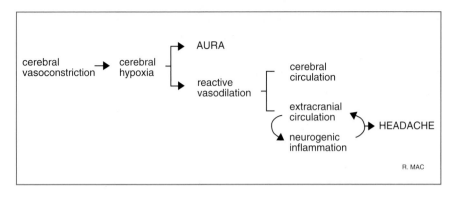

Figure 6.10. *Traditional view on the pathogenesis of the migraine attack, in which the aura and headache are considered sequential and causally related.*

In migraine without aura, as the traditional view maintains, the cerebral vasoconstriction and hypoxia occur as well but in a clinically silent area of the cerebral cortex. However, there is little evidence for this assumption and there is also no evidence that cerebral vasodilation is associated with dilation of extracranial arteries. The two assumptions were made to causally connect the migraine aura with the headache and to bring the two forms of migraine, that is, migraine with and without aura, together in one pathogenetic concept. However, on the basis of the results of the cerebral blood flow studies, it can be stated that the aura and headache are *not* causally related through cerebral vasodilation because the cerebral vasodilation, if it happens at all, does not occur until *after* the onset of the headache.

What is an alternative concept?

Except for the aura, the clinical presentations of migraine with and without aura are so similar that a common pathogenesis is plausible. Also, the two forms of migraine often occur in the same individual, with some headaches preceded, and some not, by an aura. The fact that the aura often occurs before the onset of the headache does not necessarily make it the *cause* of the headache. It is relatively simplistic reasoning to assume that because one event follows the other, there is, therefore, a causal relationship between the two.

The particular time-relationship between the occurrence of the aura and headache can also be explained in other ways. For example, with a disturbance in physiology, the reactivity of the cerebral cortex is much greater than that of the extracranial tissues in giving rise to symptoms. In the alternative concept, the pathogenesis of the migraine aura and headache are considered parallel rather than sequential in nature (Figure 6.11). They are joined together by the migraine process, the driving force behind the migraine attack. The migraine process is activated, often in unison, by the migraine triggers. There is evidence from a psychophysiological study that the visual cortex of patients with migraine *with* aura lacks inhibitory activity, in comparison to patients with migraine without aura and non-headache controls[14]. This lack of inhibitory activity could translate in hyperexcitability or a lower threshold for initiation of the spreading excitation/depression phenomenon by the migraine process. It is possible that this hyperexcitability, in turn, relates to a genetically determined calcium-channelopathy in the central nervous system[13].

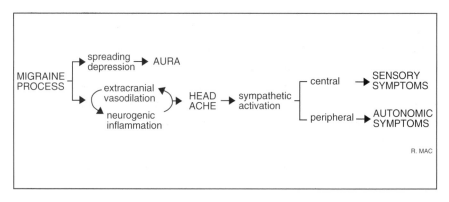

Figure 6.11. *Alternative view on the pathogenesis of the migraine attack, in which the aura and headache are considered parallel phenomena and the associated symptoms looked upon secondary to the headache. Adapted from reference 17.*

The parallel concept explains better than the sequential concept the isolated occurrence of the migraine aura (migraine aura without headache) and the isolated occurrence of the migraine headache (migraine without aura). The concept also includes the associated, autonomic and sensory symptoms of the migraine headache, explained as secondary to the headache through stimulation of the sympathetic nervous system and ascending reticular activating system, respectively.

What is the brainstem generator?

A study using positron-emission tomography showed cerebral blood flow to be increased during the migraine headache in the cingulate cortex, as well as in the visual and auditory cortices[20]. The activation of the cingulate cortex, part of the limbic system, is directly related to the pain of the migraine headache and the emotional response to it. The activation of the visual and auditory associate cortices has been related tentatively to the photophobia and phonophobia. In addition to these changes in cortical cerebral blood flow, an increase in blood flow was observed in the contralateral brainstem at the level of the mesencephalon (Figure 6.12). This change in blood flow, reflecting increased neuronal activity, was thought to be particular to migraine because it did not occur with capsaicin-induced head pain. It was also found that while administration of sumatriptan resulted in relief of the migraine symptoms and disappearance of the cortical activation, the localized increase in mesencephalic blood flow persisted. It was, therefore, suggested that the observed activation in the brainstem contralateral to the pain was the first visualization of a postulated migraine center. From this center, the above-mentioned migraine process could be initiated, activated by the migraine trigger factors.

Unfortunately, the finding of localized brainstem activation during the migraine headache has not been replicated yet, which would be the first step in solidifying its significance. Also, the brainstem area involved is thought to play an important role in central pain control rather than in the generation of pain. Furthermore, it is not known how activation of this area could cause the cerebrocortical and extracranial changes related to the migraine aura and headache, respectively. Equally obscure are the mechanisms and pathways through which this brainstem area could be activated by the diversity of trigger factors involved in migraine.

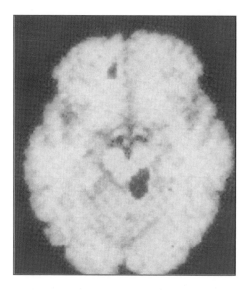

Figure 6.12. *Increased blood flow in an area of mesencephalon contralateral to the pain in patients with unilateral migraine headache (n = 9), as observed with positron-emission tomography. Also shown is the increased blood flow in the ipsilateral cingulate cortex. Reproduced from reference 20.*

CHAPTER 7

DIAGNOSIS

When should migraine be considered?

Migraine is a chronic condition of recurring headaches, which is where the diagnosis should particularly be considered. Sometimes migraine manifests itself in recurring transient focal neurological symptoms, that is, isolated migraine aura or migraine aura without headache. Therefore, the diagnosis should also be considered in cases where there is a recurrence of neurological symptoms. However, the neurological symptoms have to be sensory in nature, visual or somatosensory, and fully reversible. They typically develop slowly, that is, over minutes, and last for 10-30 minutes. They are often presented as a loss of function, for example, loss of vision or somatosensation, while, in reality, function is not lost but disturbed. Hence, the symptoms of disturbed vision are scintillations in one or both visual fields and those of disturbed somatosensation, paresthesias in one or the other side of the body.

Similar sensory symptoms are seen with focal, occipital or temporal lobe epilepsy. However, in epilepsy the symptoms progress over seconds rather than minutes and are followed by loss of consciousness, due to generalization of the seizure activity. The transient focal neurological symptoms encountered in transient ischemic attacks are different in other ways. They truly represent loss of function, come on suddenly and generally without progression, and last for seconds to minutes. The resolution of the symptoms is also different from that in migraine: in transient ischemic attacks, what is involved first, resolves last while in migraine, what is involved first, resolves first.

Case studies of migraine aura without headache

A 32-year-old woman in the final months of pregnancy experiences a visual disturbance. The disturbance consists of a shiny light close to the center of vision, which develops into a twinkling star. The star opens on the inside to give rise to a semi-circle of scintillating, gold and silver zigzag lines. The semicircle gradually expands as it moves into one of the visual fields and subsequently fades away. The visual disturbance lasts for 10-15 minutes. It is not associated with or followed by headache or any other symptom.

A 39-year-old woman has experienced a visual disturbance for two years. The disturbance starts with a cloud appearing in front of the left eye. After five minutes, a bowed line of bright and flickering zigzag lines appears in the upper quadrant of the left visual field. The bowed line, which gives the impression of being electrified, disappears after 30 minutes as abruptly as it starts. She has the visual disturbance once per month and feels completely exhausted afterward but without headache.

The transient focal neurological symptoms of migraine are different from those of epilepsy and transient ischemic attacks.

Case study of temporal lobe epilepsy

A 23-year-old woman experiences fear of entering supermarkets because she fainted twice while shopping in one. Prior to the fainting, she experienced tingling, which lasted for seconds and moved very rapidly from the right hand into the lower arm and shoulder. She subsequently lost consciousness and woke up, lying on the floor. She did not bite her tongue or loose urine. Electroencephalography and cranial computerized tomography with contrast were normal.

Case study of transient ischemic attacks

A 47-year-old man experiences two types of attacks. The first type consists of loss of feeling in the right hand and forearm, which comes on in 10 seconds. The loss of feeling is associated with weakness and clumsiness. The attacks occur two or three times per week and last for two to five minutes. He has experienced them for four to five months. The second type of attack consists of a loss of peripheral vision in the left eye. The loss of vision is concentric and gray rather than black. It develops in 5-10 minutes and lasts for 15-30 minutes. This type of attack he has experienced for three weeks. On examination, he has a high-pitch bruit in the neck over the left carotid artery. Angiography revealed a stenosis of more than 90% at the origin of the left internal carotid artery (Figure 7.1).

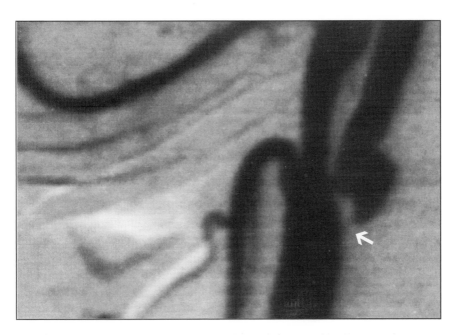

Figure 7.1. *Carotid angiogram of a patient with transient ischemic attacks, showing a more than 90% stenosis at the origin of the left internal carotid artery (arrow).*

Should migraine be considered in acute, severe headache?

The diagnosis of migraine in acute, severe headache should be considered only if there is a prior history of similar headaches. In the presence of fever, meningitis, either viral or bacterial, is an important differential diagnosis to take into account. Meningitis occurs mostly before age 20 years and is particularly important to consider in a child with acute, severe headache. A patient with bacterial meningitis is generally very sick and can be delirious. The headache of viral meningitis, on the other hand, can easily be mistaken for a migraine headache. In meningitis, examination will reveal limited forward flexion of the neck with intact rotation. The diagnosis is made through lumbar puncture, which should be performed in every patient in whom the condition is suspected.

Acute, severe headache without fever is suspicious for intracranial hemorrhage, especially subarachnoid hemorrhage. The headache caused by intracranial hemorrhage has a very sudden onset and comes on in a matter of seconds, like a blow to the head. In a patient with acute, severe headache, the onset of headache is, therefore, always very important to establish as precisely as possible. The headache of migraine comes on relatively slowly and requires several hours to build to its maximum intensity. The headache of cluster headache builds to its maximum intensity more rapidly but still requires 5-10 minutes.

Subarachnoid hemorrhage occurs in particular in the age group of 20-50 years, which is also when migraine is most common. The importance of diagnosing subarachnoid hemorrhage lies in the fact that it is still associated with a mortality rate as high as 50%. In subarachnoid hemorrhage, as in meningitis, examination will reveal limited forward flexion of the neck with intact rotation. The diagnosis is made through computerized tomography without contrast or, if the scan is negative or the test not available, through lumbar puncture. As with meningitis, the diagnostic tests, including lumbar puncture if indicated, should be performed in every suspected patient.

Case study of meningitis

A 17-year-old man experiences severe headache, which has been present for one day. The headache started around noontime and gradually increased in intensity. He went to sleep at night but it woke him up at 2a.m. The headache is associated with photophobia, nausea, vomiting, and diarrhea. He also feels off balance and cannot walk straight. The headache is located across the forehead and throbbing in nature. It is made worse by coughing and bending over, while ice applied to the forehead makes it somewhat better. He does not have fever but has felt hot and cold; his sister was sick with the flu. On examination, he is clearly sick with headache and nausea. His fundi cannot be examined because of extreme photophobia. It is slightly difficult to bend his neck forward. A lumbar puncture revealed clear and colorless fluid, which contained 380 cells per mm^3 of which 90% were lymphocytes, indicating viral meningitis.

Case study of subarachnoid hemorrhage

A 56-year-old woman experiences severe headache, which started the night before during intercourse. According to her husband, she suddenly grasped her head and, for a short moment, was dazed. After she took an analgesic, she fell asleep. However, in the morning he had a hard time waking her up. The headache was still severe and she vomited several times. Her husband had to support her, while walking downstairs because she could not see the steps. On examination, she looks sick and is slightly drowsy. She has a severe headache, radiating up from the neck into the forehead, with pressure in the eyes. Her temperature is normal and the fundi show sharply defined optic disks, without hemorrhage. However, her neck is difficult to bend forward while rotation is intact. She also bends her knees when the neck is bent forward. Cranial computerized tomography without contrast was unremarkable but lumbar puncture revealed hemorrhagic fluid, which was yellow after centrifugation. Angiography showed an aneurysm of the left posterior communicating artery (Figure 7.2).

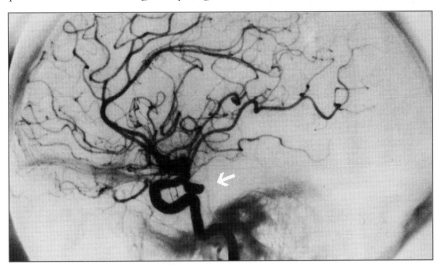

Figure 7.2. *Carotid angiogram, showing an aneurysm (arrow) of the left posterior communicating artery in a patient with subarachnoid hemorrhage. Reproduced from reference 1.*

What are the diagnostic features of migraine?

Recurring headaches of moderate or severe intensity is the most important diagnostic feature of migraine. In between the headaches, the patient is symptom-free and this should be ascertained in the history. If headaches do occur frequently in between the migraine headaches, chronic migraine should be considered. Migraine headaches occur at a greatly varying frequency from once per year to once or twice per week. However, when the headaches occur frequently, that is, once per week or more, chronic migraine should again be considered. Also the duration of migraine headaches varies greatly but is minimally four to six hours, although it can be shorter in children. According to the diagnostic criteria of the International Headache Society, the maximum duration of the migraine headache is 72 hours, after which it is referred to as status migrainosus or migraine status. However, a migraine headache can continue for several days and still end by itself, which is particularly seen in menstrual migraine.

The migraine headache comes on during the day or is present on awakening in the morning. It sometimes wakes the patient up out of sleep at night, usually in the early hours of the morning, between 4.a.m. and 6a.m. Only the headache of cluster headache wakes the patient up out of sleep in the early hours of the night, between midnight and 2a.m. The migraine headache can be present in its full intensity on awakening in the morning or when it wakes the patient up out of sleep at night. Otherwise, it generally requires at least one to two hours to build to its maximum intensity.

What are other features of the migraine headache?

In two-thirds of patients, the migraine headache is limited to one side of the head. Typically the headache alternates between the two sides, although often with a preference for one particular side. When the headache *always* occurs on the same side, that is, when it is fixed in its lateralization, further investigation is required. It may reveal a structural intracranial lesion, as in so-called symptomatic migraine, or another type of lateralized abnormality of the head, face, or neck.

Case study of unilateral sinusitis causing fixed lateralization

A 46-year-old woman has experienced headaches since her early twenties. The headaches occur three or four times per month, especially perimenstrually. They are present on awakening in the morning and build to their maximum intensity in four to six hours. The headaches are moderate or severe in intensity and last for one to six days. They are located in the right side of the forehead and are sharp, steady in nature. The headaches are sometimes associated with nausea but never with photophobia or phonophobia. She also experiences bifrontal headaches that are mild in intensity. These headaches occur two or three times per week. They come on around noontime and last for the remainder of the day. She also has nasal congestion, especially of the right nostril, associated with postnasal drip. Cranial magnetic-resonance imaging revealed chronic maxillary sinusitis on the right (Figure 7.3). Surgical treatment resulted in a decrease in the frequency of the bifrontal headaches; the right-sided headaches improved as well and now alternate sides.

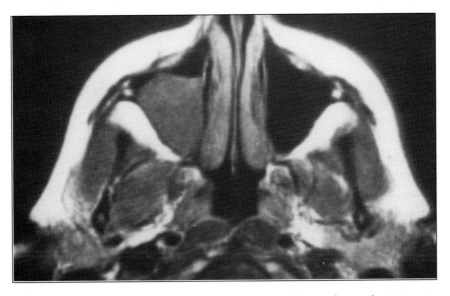

Figure 7.3. *Cranial magnetic-resonance scan, T1-weighted transverse image, showing chronic maxillary sinusitis on the right in a patient with right-sided migraine headaches.*

Case study of unilateral neck spasm causing fixed lateralization

A 43-year-old woman has experienced headaches since age 16. The headaches occur monthly with menstruation and last for three to four days. They are present on awakening in the morning and are severe in intensity. The headaches feel like a pressure behind the left eye, as if the eye is being pushed out of the socket. They are associated with nausea, vomiting, photophobia, and blurred vision in the left eye. In addition to the headaches, the left back of the neck is always very tight and sore, related to spasm of the neck muscles. She has had the neck muscle spasm as long as she remembers. At times of stress or fatigue, the spasm is worse and causes headache. Physical therapy and trigger-point injections decreased the muscle spasm, as a result of which the headaches became alternating.

MIGRAINE

The migraine headache is often localized, generally in the temple, eye, or forehead but sometimes in the back of the head. It is typically dull, throbbing or sharp, steady in nature and made worse by physical activity, such as walking up a flight of stairs, bending over, straining, coughing, *etc.* Lying down still in a dark and quiet room – sometimes with the head slightly elevated – can improve the headache somewhat. Also, applying pressure on the temple(s) or a cold cloth over the forehead often provides some temporary relief.

The migraine headache is almost always associated with other symptoms, of which the gastrointestinal ones are the most prominent, ranging from lack of appetite to vomiting. There is generally also increased sensitivity of the sensory organs in terms of photophobia, phonophobia, and osmophobia. The photophobia and phonophobia can be so intense that exposure to light or noise actually aggravates the intensity of the pain. The osmophobia is often connected with the gastrointestinal symptoms, which are, consequently, made worse by exposure to a strong smell or odor.

What are chronic and transformed migraine?

In chronic migraine, headaches occur daily or almost daily in association with migraine headaches, which generally occur frequently, sometimes as often as several times per week. However, the patients often present themselves as having intermittent headaches, while most of them actually have a continuous headache. This is important to recognize early in the taking of the history because it necessitates a different approach. With daily headaches, the emphasis should be on the daily headaches, which should also be the focus of the treatment[2]. Once the daily headaches improve, the severe migraine headaches generally follow suit.

In clinical practice, more than 90% of the patients with daily headaches have also migraine headaches[4]. In the general population, about half of those afflicted with daily headaches have migraine headaches. In practice, a quarter of the patients with chronic migraine has severe headaches more than 15 days per month. These are the patients that tend to be most disabled as a result of their headaches. Two-third of the patients develop the daily headaches gradually out of initially intermittent headaches and one-third develop them abruptly[5]. The initially intermittent headaches are tension-type in one-third and migraine in two-third[6]. When the chronic migraine condition gradually develops out of intermittent migraine headaches, it is also referred to as transformed migraine. The fact that both (episodic) tension-type headache and migraine can progress to the same daily headache condition is the basis for the tension-migraine headache continuum, shown in Figure 7.4. The progression of episodic tension-type headache to daily headaches results first in chronic tension-type headache, before migraine headaches are added to the presentation.

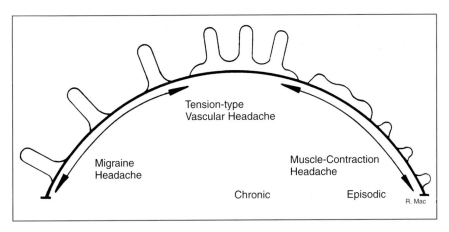

Figure 7.4. *The tension-migraine headache continuum, showing the interrelationship of episodic and chronic tension-type headache and episodic and chronic migraine. When the chronic migraine condition develops out of episodic migraine, it is also referred to as transformed migraine.*

Case study of daily headache developed out of migraine

A 41-year-old woman has experienced headaches since her late teens. Initially, the headaches occurred once per week and lasted for 24 hours. They were severe in intensity and sometimes associated with nausea and vomiting. Over time, the headaches gradually increased in frequency and became daily 15 years ago. The daily headaches are present on awakening in the morning or wake her up out of sleep at night. They are generally worst in the morning on awakening and get somewhat better as the day progresses. The headaches start in the back of the neck and extend forward into both temples and sometimes also into the left eye. They are throbbing in nature in the temples and sharp, steady in the eye. The headaches are severe two or three times per month for 48 hours. The severe headaches are associated with nausea, vomiting, photophobia, and phonophobia. Stress and exertion make the headaches worse and they are also worse premenstrually.

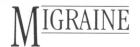

In addition to the headaches, she has very tight and sore neck and shoulder muscles, especially on the left.

Case study of daily headache developed out of tension-type headache

A 44-year-old woman has experienced headaches since her late teens or early twenties. Initially, the headaches occurred once per week. They came on in the late afternoon and lasted for several hours. The headaches were mild in intensity, located across the forehead, and not associated with other symptoms. Over time, they gradually increased in frequency and intensity and became daily five years ago. The daily headaches are present on awakening in the morning three days per week or come on in the afternoon. They gradually increase in intensity as the day progresses and are worst in the evening. The headaches rarely wake her up out of sleep at night. They are located across the forehead, giving a feeling of tightness, except when severe. They are severe once or twice per month for three to four days. The severe headaches are located in the sides of the head and throbbing in nature. They are associated with nausea, photophobia, and phonophobia. The severe headaches particularly occur with menstruation and, to a lesser extent, with ovulation. The neck muscles are always very tight and sore, equally on both sides.

What is the evidence for the tension-migraine headache continuum?

On the tension-migraine headache continuum, we find episodic and chronic tension-type headache and episodic and chronic migraine. Episodic tension-type headache is experienced almost universally, while episodic migraine affects approximately 12% of the population 12-80 years old. Of the chronic headache conditions, chronic tension-type headache affects approximately 3% of the population and the same is true for chronic migraine. In comparison, cluster headache affects approximately 0.1% of the population. The major distinction between tension-type headache and migraine is the intensity of the headaches. Headache intensity is generally divided into three categories, mild, moderate, and severe, depending on the extent to which the headache affects the ability to function. A mild headache does not affect the ability to function, a moderate headache affects the ability to function but does not necessitate bed rest, and a severe headache is incapacitating and requires bed rest.

Tension-type headaches are mild or moderate in intensity and migraine headaches are generally moderate or severe, but can be mild. Related to the intensity of the pain, tension-type headaches have few, if any, symptoms associated with them and when symptoms are present, they are mild. Migraine headaches, on the other hand, have intense associated symptoms related to the high intensity of the pain. Almost universally present in migraine are photophobia and phonophobia; however, also nausea is common and with the most intense migraine headaches, vomiting occurs as well.

The concept of the tension-migraine headache continuum is supported by the results of a study of patients with daily headaches I conducted in my practice[3]. The study involved 258 patients, 50 men and 208 women, who experienced headaches at least five days per week for at least one year. Only those patients who had so-called paroxysmal daily headaches, that is, cluster headache or paroxysmal hemicrania, were excluded from the study. At the time of consultation, the average age of the patients was slightly over 40; more than 75% of them had experienced the onset of headaches before age 30 years. The onset was more common in the second decade of life in women then in men (36 *versus* 24%), compatible with the importance the onset of menstruation has on headache in women.

In the study, 37% of the patients abruptly developed the daily headaches and 63% developed them gradually out of initially intermittent headaches. Of the latter group, 33% initially experienced mild headaches and 67% severe headaches. The mild headaches were in 25% associated with nausea but never with vomiting, while the severe headaches were in 84% associated with nausea and in 72% with vomiting. The mild headaches were, therefore, compatible with the diagnosis of episodic tension-type headache and the severe headaches with migraine. However, the features of the daily headaches that these patients ultimately developed were the same, whether the initial headaches were mild or severe in intensity. The features looked at in the study were diurnal headache pattern, nocturnal headache awakening, laterality and associated symptoms of the daily headaches, occurrence of severe headaches, and frequency, laterality, and associated symptoms of the severe headaches. The transition from intermittent into daily headaches in the patients studied was truly gradual and, on average, took a decade (Figure 7.5).

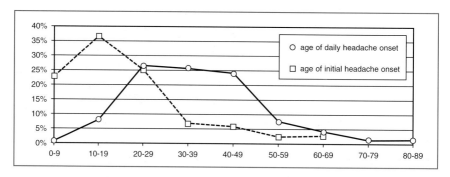

Figure 7.5. *Distribution of the age of onset of the initial and daily headaches in the patients, who gradually developed the daily headaches out of initially intermittent headaches (n = 106 and 145, respectively). Reproduced from reference 6.*

Of the 145 patients who gradually developed the daily headaches out of initially intermittent headaches, 91 could be contacted for follow-up. Of these patients, 23 or 25% still had daily headaches. Of the remaining 68 patients with intermittent headaches, 46 were able to provide enough information to allow the diagnosis of their initial, intermittent headaches. Of these patients, 39 or 85% initially had episodic migraine and seven or 15% initially had episodic tension-type headache. Of the 39 patients who initially had episodic migraine, then gradually developed daily headaches, and now again experienced intermittent headaches, 77% now also had migraine and 23% tension-type headache. The group of patients who initially had episodic tension-type headache, then gradually developed daily headaches, and now again experienced intermittent headaches, was too small to analyze.

On the basis of the study, it can be stated that with progression from intermittent to daily headaches, the daily headache condition is the same whether the initial headaches are tension-type or migraine. With reversal back to intermittent headaches, the majority of the patients who initially had migraine went back to having migraine headaches, a finding also in support of the headache continuum presented.

What is symptomatic migraine?

Symptomatic migraine, also called migraine mimic, is a condition caused by structural neurological illness, manifesting itself as migraine. As migraine is a chronic condition, the structural neurological illnesses that cause symptomatic migraine are either not progressive or progress very slowly. Arteriovenous malformation and meningioma are examples of such conditions that can manifest themselves as migraine. Fixed and crossed lateralization of the headaches and the neurological symptoms or signs is a feature to look for as an indication of symptomatic migraine. This means that the headaches *always* occur on the same side and the neurological symptoms or signs *always* on the opposite side. Another feature to look for is the persistence of neurological symptoms or signs in between the headaches.

Case study of symptomatic migraine caused by meningioma

A 33-year-old woman has experienced headaches for seven years. Initially, the headaches occurred infrequently and were mild in intensity. Over time, they gradually increased in frequency and intensity and have been almost daily for the last year. The daily headaches usually come on around noontime and are worse in the late afternoon or early evening. They are generally located in the right forehead but sometimes are bilateral in location. The headaches are not associated with nausea, vomiting, photophobia, or phonophobia. Cranial computerized tomography with contrast revealed a frontoparietal meningioma on the right (Figure 7.6).

MIGRAINE

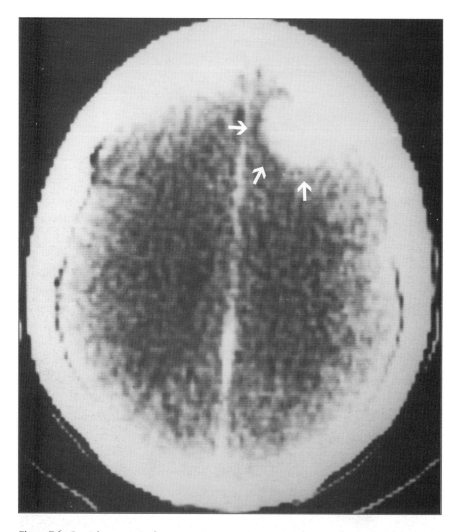

Figure 7.6. *Cranial computerized tomogram transverse contrast, axial image, showing a meningioma on the right (arrows) in a patient with symptomatic migraine without aura. Reproduced from reference 1.*

Case study of symptomatic migraine caused by arteriovenous malformation

A 37-year-old man has experienced headaches since college. Until five years ago, the headaches had occurred once per month and after that, two or three times per year.

However, over the last 10 days he has experienced the headaches five times. The headaches come on during the day, usually in the afternoon. They build to their maximum intensity in 5-10 minutes and last for 6-12 hours. The headaches are located on the left, in the forehead and behind the eye. They feel like an intense pressure and in half of them, the pain is severe. The headaches are associated with photophobia and occasionally

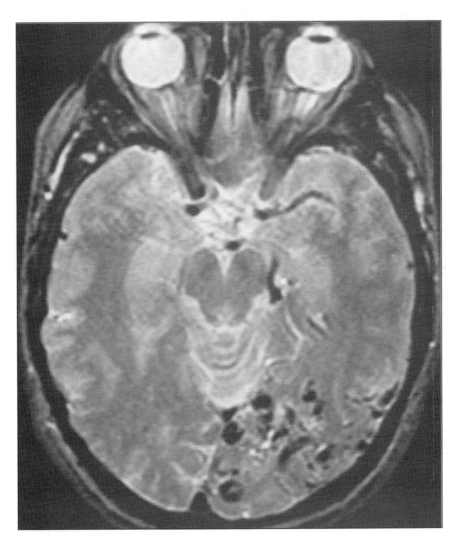

Figure 7.7. *Cranial magnetic-resonance scan, T1-weighted transverse image showing a large arteriovenous malformation of the left occipital lobe in a patient with symptomatic migraine with aura.*

also with nausea and vomiting. They are preceded for 10-20 minutes by a visual disturbance, consisting of blue spots in the right visual field. The visual disturbance lasts for the duration of the headache. Bright light, overexertion, red wine, monosodium glutamate, and more than two cups of coffee bring on headache. Cranial magnetic-resonance imaging revealed a large arteriovenous malformation of the left occipital lobe (Figure 7.7).

CHAPTER 8

ABORTIVE TREATMENT

When is abortive migraine treatment indicated?

Abortive treatment of migraine is *always* indicated because the headaches are so intense that they interfere with the ability to function. However, not only the headache, through its intensity, causes disability; the associated gastrointestinal symptoms contribute as well. In actual fact, it is often the nausea and vomiting that force the patient to lie down because motion and activity tend to aggravate these symptoms.

The goal of abortive migraine treatment is to provide *full* relief of symptoms within two hours of initiation of treatment. Only then can the treatment be considered effective and we currently have the (pharmacological) tools to accomplish this for most patients. Effective abortive treatment is important from a humanistic as well as public-health perspective. From a humanistic perspective, it is important because of the suffering migraine involves and the strain it places on personal relationships and professional development. From a public-health perspective, it is important because *in*effective abortive treatment facilitates the progression of the condition, ultimately leading to chronic migraine. The progression is often attributed to overuse of abortive medications; however, with the exception of vasoconstrictors, ineffective treatment may be more so the culprit. Effective treatment has the additional benefit of decreasing headache recurrence, as shown in Figure 8.1 for frovatriptan and naratriptan.

Abortive treatment aims at decreasing the intensity of the headache, if possible, to its full relief. Effective reduction in headache intensity generally also leads to relief of the associated symptoms, nausea, vomiting, photophobia, and phonophobia. The gastrointestinal symptoms can also be addressed separately with antinausea medications, such as metoclopramide or domperidone. There is no specific treatment for the sensory symptoms, that is, photophobia and phonophobia, but accommodating the patient in a dark and quiet room may relieve them.

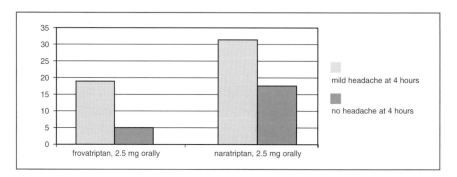

Figure 8.1. *Recurrence of moderate or severe headache within 24 hours of treatment with frovatriptan, 2.5 mg orally, or naratriptan, 2.5 mg orally, as a function of headache relief at 4 hours after treatment. Frovatriptan data obtained from reference 16 and naratriptan data obtained from reference 11.*

Lying down, sometimes with the head elevated, often also decreases the intensity of the pain and, therefore, can reduce the nausea and vomiting as well. A cold compress applied to the head, especially to the forehead and temples, and sometimes putting pressure on the temples, can also help decrease the intensity of the pain.

What are the approaches to the abortive treatment of migraine?

The three approaches to the abortive treatment of migraine are step care, stratified care, and staged care. In *step care*, treatment is initiated with the least potent medication, either acetaminophen or a non-steroidal anti-inflammatory analgesic, like aspirin. If ineffective, a mild vasoconstrictor is added, such as caffeine or isometheptene. A next step up is to add codeine or barbiturate to the combination or to change to a relatively strong opioid, such as hydrocodone or oxycodone. A further increase in potency is to prescribe an oral triptan and as further steps up, an intranasal and subcutaneous triptan. As alternatives to the intranasal and subcutaneous triptan, an intranasal and rectal or subcutaneous ergot, respectively, can be used. Clearly, step care is a cumbersome approach that requires time and patience from the patient and physician alike. Eventually, both parties may become so frustrated with the process that treatment is abandoned before it is completed.

In *stratified* care, an assessment is made of the ultimate intensity of the headaches and treatment is chosen accordingly. For example, mild headaches are treated with acetaminophen or a non-steroidal anti-inflammatory analgesic, moderate headaches with an analgesic combination containing caffeine or isometheptene, and severe headaches with (the addition of) an opioid analgesic, triptan, or ergot. The problem with this approach is that oral medications are relied upon and the impaired functioning of the gastrointestinal tract during the migraine headache is not taken into account. This impaired gastrointestinal functioning results in atony and dilation of the stomach with closure of the pyloric sphincter[8] (Figure 8.2). It causes a delay in gastric emptying, which has been shown to correlate highly with the intensity of the pain[1] ($r_s = 0.84$; $p<0.01$). The final outcome of the delayed gastric emptying is a decrease in absorption of medications taken orally, including some of the triptans (Figure 8.3).

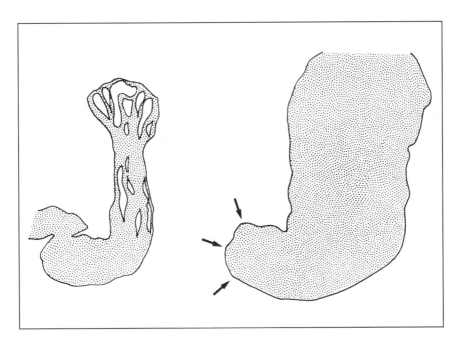

Figure 8.2. *Upper gastrointestinal tract between and during migraine headaches, showing atony and dilation of the stomach with closure of the pyloric sphincter (arrows) during the headache. Drawn on the basis of reference 8.*

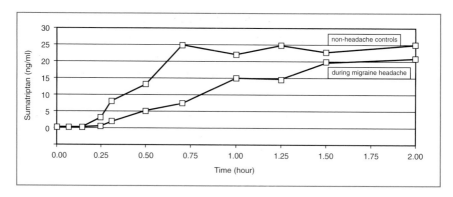

Figure 8.3. *Plasma levels of sumatriptan, as a function of time, after administration of 50 mg orally in non-headache controls (n = 26) and during migraine headache (n = 26). Adapted from reference 10.*

Gastrokinetic medications, which stimulate the activity of the gastrointestinal tract, have been shown to improve the impaired absorption of medications taken orally during migraine headache[20]. The medications available in this category are metoclopramide and domperidone. The additional advantage of these medications is that they do not cause drowsiness and effectively relieve nausea and vomiting. The absence of drowsiness is important because in order to be beneficial, they have to be taken at mild headache intensity to be absorbed themselves. Once in the system, they limit the impairment of gastrointestinal functioning during migraine headache that occurs with increasing pain intensity. The gastrokinetic medications also mitigate the occurrence of nausea and vomiting, which results from the abnormal gastrointestinal functioning as well. This strategy, however, only works when the patient is in the position to treat the migraine headaches at mild pain intensity. This is only possible when the headaches come on during the day and increase in intensity gradually, allowing early treatment. When taken very early, if possible before the onset of the headache, the gastrokinetic medications may have the additional benefit of preventing further development of the attack. This has been shown for domperidone[21] and I have observed a similar effect with metoclopramide[12]. Treatment of the headache *per se* should be initiated shortly after intake of the gastrokinetic medication, not to allow the pain to become too intense.

The above-described gastrointestinal changes of the migraine headache are taken into account in *staged care*, which makes it the most optimal of the three approaches. In staged care, the choice of treatment is based on the intensity of the headache *at the time of treatment.* Migraine headaches often develop in a certain pattern and patients can generally describe the typical mode of onset of their headaches. An important question to ask is whether the headaches usually come on during the day, are present on awakening in the morning, or wake the patient up out of sleep at night. In case the headaches typically are present on awakening in the morning or wake the patient up out of sleep at night, their intensity should be assessed at that point. The patient can use a 3- or 10-point scale to rate the intensity of the headaches. The 3-point scale rates the pain as mild, moderate, or severe, depending on the extent to which the headaches affect the ability to function. A mild headache does not affect the ability to function, a moderate headache affects the ability to function but does not necessitate bed rest, and a severe headache is incapacitating and requires bed rest. The 10-point scale goes from no pain (0) to the most excruciating pain imaginable to the patient (10). If the headache comes on during the day, the question is how long it takes for the headache to build to its maximum intensity.

After the above information has been obtained for the typical migraine headache, it is important to know how often headaches come on or develop differently and, if they do, in what way. It then needs to be decided whether one strategy can be relied upon or whether the patient should also be given a second, rescue strategy, in case the first treatment fails.

What kinds of medications can be used for abortive treatment of the headache?

For the abortive treatment of the migraine headache, three types of medications can be used: analgesics, antiphlogistics, that is, anti-inflammatory medications, and vasoconstrictors (Table 8.1). The antiphlogistics and vasoconstrictors are more specific for the migraine headache, addressing the mechanisms of neurogenic inflammation and arterial vasodilation, respectively. As a result, they are generally more effective and, therefore, preferred. The analgesics, acetaminophen and the opioids, tend to be relatively ineffective because they solely address the pain. In addition, the opioids are absorbed relatively poorly when given orally and can be addicting. Migraine is a chronic and often, life-long condition and, therefore, the use of potentially addicting medications should be avoided, if possible. The antiphlogistics include aspirin and the non-steroidal anti-inflammatory analgesics. The vasoconstrictors can be divided into three groups, that is, caffeine, sympathomimetics, and serotoninergics and the serotoninergics, in turn, can be divided into selective and non-selective.

Table 8.1. *Categories of medications for the abortive treatment of the migraine headache*

Analgesics		
	Acetaminophen	
	Opioids	
Antiphlogistics = non-steroidal		
anti-inflammatory analgesics		
Vasoconstrictors	Caffeine	
	Sympathomimetics	
	Serotoninergics	
		Selective = triptans
		Non-selective = ergots

Caffeine is the vasoconstrictor that is used most commonly, either alone, as in a strong cup of coffee, a home remedy for headache, or in combination with other medications. In combination with analgesics, it has been shown to increase their potency by 40%[9]. Apart from having itself some analgesic effect, it improves the absorption of medications with which it is combined. However, it is often not realized that caffeine is relatively long acting and may remain in the system for up to 60 hours, which is almost three days! Therefore, it should not be used for the abortive treatment of headache, including migraine, more often than two to three days per week. If used more frequently, it accumulates in the system and causes headache whenever its effect wears off, creating a vascular rebound cycle. This is also an important mechanism by which headaches, over time, increase in frequency and ultimately become daily.

Analgesics are, either alone or in combination with caffeine, only moderately effective in the abortive treatment of migraine headaches.

However, combining them with a gastrokinetic medication, such as metoclopramide or domperidone, often increases their efficacy. These gastrokinetic medications have the unique property of stimulating the activity of the gastrointestinal tract and, in addition, effectively relieve nausea.

Of the non-steroidal anti-inflammatory analgesics, aspirin is used most commonly, either alone or in combination with caffeine, metoclopramide, or both. Since they became available without prescription, ibuprofen, ketoprofen, and naproxen sodium have been used more often as well. The stomach generally tolerates these non-steroidal anti-inflammatory analgesics better than aspirin, with less heartburn and pain. However, the medications need to be given in relatively high doses in order to be effective. They may also be effective only when given at mild pain intensity and after pre-treatment with a gastrokinetic medication. Indomethacin is a non-steroidal anti-inflammatory analgesic that deserves special mention because it is not only a potent analgesic and anti-inflammatory medication but also a constrictor of the cranial arteries. However, it is not absorbed well orally and, therefore, should be prescribed as a rectal suppository, which comes in doses of 50 and 100 mg.

Which are the vasoconstrictors other than caffeine?

The vasoconstrictors are divided into sympathomimetics and serotoninergics. The sympathomimetic vasoconstrictors release catecholamines from the sympathetic nerve terminals or directly stimulate postsynaptic α-adrenoceptors. The sympathomimetic vasoconstrictors are mostly used as decongestants, for example, phenylephrine, a directly acting sympathomimetic. In the United States, an indirectly acting sympathomimetic, called isometheptene, is also available for the abortive treatment of migraine headaches.

The serotoninergic vasoconstrictors are more potent than the sympathomimetic ones and include the triptans and ergots. The triptans are more selective in their mode of action than the ergots and, as a result, have fewer side effects and are safer to use. In addition, they are absorbed better, especially when given orally. Ergotamine is the oldest of the serotoninergic vasoconstrictors and was introduced into the treatment of migraine in 1926. Its potent constrictor effect on the extracranial (temporal and occipital) arteries in man is shown in Figure 8.4. Ergotamine also has an effect on neurogenic inflammation, which is illustrated in Figure 8.5 in relation to its effect on the intensity of the migraine headache.

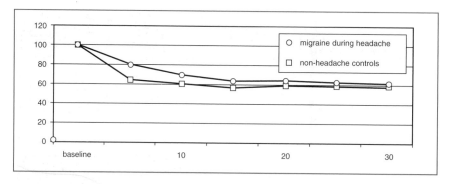

Figure 8.4. *Percentage decrease in pulsation amplitude of the extracranial (temporal and occipital) arteries during migraine headache (n = 20) and in non-headache controls (n = 34), after intravenous administration of 0.37-0.5 mg ergotamine. Data obtained from reference 6.*

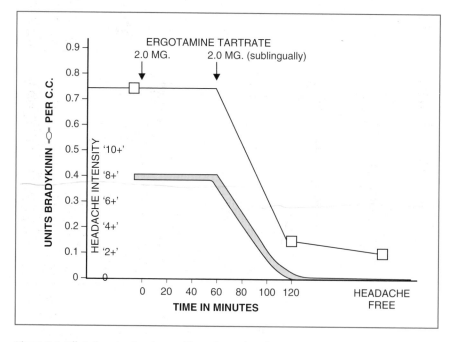

Figure 8.5. *Effect of ergotamine, 4 mg sublingually, on the inflammatory activity of subcutaneous perfusates of sites of migraine headache, in bradykinin units, in relation to the effect on the intensity of the pain. Reproduced from reference 2.*

The gastrointestinal absorption of ergotamine is better when combined with caffeine and the medication is available in that combination as a tablet and rectal suppository[5].

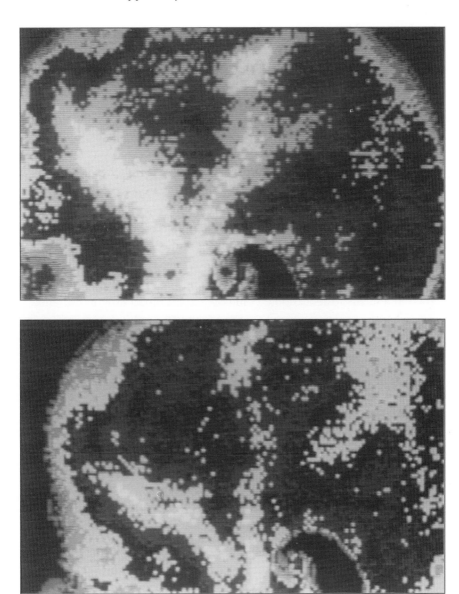

Figure 8.6. *Thermograms of the lateral side of the head, showing the superficial temporal artery in white before above and 30 minutes after intravenous administration of 0.5 mg dihydroergotamine below.*

A derivative of ergotamine, dihydroergotamine, was introduced into the abortive treatment of migraine in 1945. It is available for parenteral administration and in the United States also as a nasal spray. Its pharmacology is very similar to that of ergotamine with quantitative rather than qualitative differences. It is four times less potent as a vasoconstrictor but ten times less potent as an emetic agent and is, therefore, better tolerated with less gastrointestinal side effects. The potent vasoconstrictor effect of dihydroergotamine on the superficial temporal artery in man is shown in Figure 8.6.

The triptans were developed in the 1980s and 90s on the basis of the vascular mode of action of the ergots. The first triptan that became available on the market was sumatriptan. Contrary to general belief, sumatriptan was *not* developed specifically for the treatment of migraine but as a pharmacological tool. It was developed as a selective agonist of the serotonin 1-like receptor that mediates contraction of the dog saphenous vein, in order to distinguish it from the serotonin 1-like receptor that mediates relaxation of the cat saphenous vein[14]. The selective serotonin 1-like receptor agonist, 5-carboxamide tryptamine, had been shown in animals to redistribute common carotid blood flow in the same way, as had been demonstrated for the ergots. The redistribution of carotid blood flow by the ergots was not due to the mere reduction they cause in carotid blood flow but to their potent constrictor effect on arteriovenous anastomoses[17]. On the basis of measurements of the oxygen saturation of blood drawn from the external jugular vein and an artery, it had been postulated that dihydroergotamine aborts migraine headaches by constricting arteriovenous anastomoses[7]. This is what established the link between the serotonin 1-like receptor, particularly the one mediating contraction of the isolated dog saphenous vein, and migraine. It was this link, rather than the observations made in the 1960s that linked serotonin and migraine, which led to the introduction of sumatriptan and, thereby, of the triptans in the abortive treatment of migraine.

The triptans, as is shown in Figure 8.7 for rizatriptan, sumatriptan, and zolmitriptan, constrict the superficial temporal artery in man. In addition, they have been demonstrated to inhibit the release of calcitonin gene-related peptide, the neuropeptide that mediates the vasodilation component of neurogenic inflammation, as is shown in Figure 8.8 for sumatriptan. There are presently seven triptans but not all of them are available on the market yet, either in Europe or the United States.

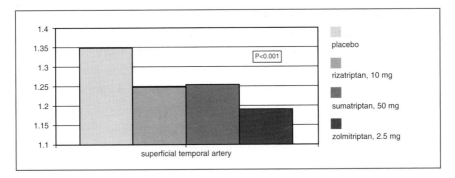

Figure 8.7. *Effect of oral triptans, 1.5-2.5 hours after administration, in comparison to placebo, on the luminal diameter of the superficial temporal artery, in mm, between migraine headaches (n = 16). Data obtained from reference 3.*

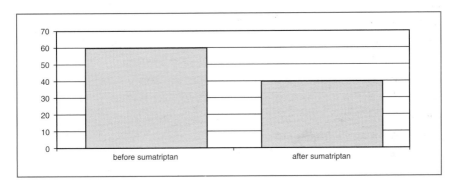

Figure 8.8. *Effect of sumatriptan, 3 or 6 mg subcutaneously, on the level of calcitonin gene-related peptide in blood drawn from the external jugular vein, in pmol/l, during migraine headaches (n = 8). Data obtained from reference 4.*

Which are the seven triptans?

The seven triptans are almotriptan, eletriptan, frovatriptan, naratriptan, rizatriptan, sumatriptan, and zolmitriptan. They are better tolerated and safer than the ergots because they are more selective in their mode of action. The triptans have affinity in particular for the serotonin 1B and 1D receptors, while the ergots also potently bind to the serotonin 1A and 2A receptors as well as to the α-adrenergic and dopaminergic receptors. Through stimulation of the serotonin 1A and dopaminergic receptors, the ergots cause nausea and vomiting. Through stimulation of the serotonin

2A receptors, they cause coronary vasoconstriction and through stimulation of the a-adrenoceptors, peripheral vasoconstriction. Their interaction with the serotonin 2A receptors makes the ergots less safe than the triptans from a cardiac perspective. The interaction with the other receptors has bearing on the tolerability of the ergots, in particular accounting for the gastrointestinal side effects and cold feet or leg cramps that can occur with their use. Nevertheless, despite their receptor selectivity, the triptans are considered contraindicated for patients with coronary artery disease or uncontrolled hypertension.

What are the optimum doses of the triptans?

Optimum-dose determination is important in the practice of medicine because the physician needs to know what dose to prescribe. This is especially true when a medication is available in more-than-one strength and can be given in a range of doses. The determination of the optimum dose is based on the results of randomized, double-blind, placebo-controlled, dose-range studies. The optimum doses of the triptans along with their tablet strengths and maximum daily doses are presented in Table 8.2.

Table 8.2. *Tablet strengths, optimum and maximum daily doses of the triptans*

Generic name	Tablet strengths	Optimum dose	Maximum daily dose
Almotriptan	6.25 and 12.5 mg	12.5 mg	25 mg
Eletriptan	20 and 40 mg	20 mg	80 mg
Frovatriptan	2.5 mg	2.5 mg	7.5 mg
Naratriptan	2.5 mg	2.5 mg	5 mg
Rizatriptan	5 and 10 mg	10 mg*	30 mg*
Sumatriptan	25, 50, and 100 mg	50 mg	200 mg
Zolmitriptan	2.5 and 5 mg	2.5 mg	10 mg

in patients on propranolol, 5 and 15 mg, respectively

The two criteria that have been applied in the optimum-dose determination of the triptans are[13]:

1. The *highest* dose that is effective and is associated with a numerical occurrence of side effects similar to placebo; and

2. The lowest dose that provides maximum therapeutic benefit where the effect levels off at a certain dose point.

For almotriptan and naratriptan, the optimum dose is the highest effective dose with placebo-level side effects; for frovatriptan, rizatriptan, and zolmitriptan, it is the lowest effective dose with maximum therapeutic benefit. Sumatriptan is the only triptan for which the optimum dose fulfills both criteria. When the above criteria are applied to eletriptan, the optimum dose that emerges is 20 mg, which is the highest effective dose with placebo-level side effects[15]. The optimum dose of a triptan can generally be repeated every two to four hours, with a maximum of two to four tablets per day.

All seven triptans are available in regular oral-tablet form. Rizatriptan and zolmitriptan are also available in orally disintegrating tablets of equal strengths, which dissolve in the mouth. Sumatriptan is also available as a nasal spray, suppository, and subcutaneous injections. The dose of the nasal spray is 20 mg and that of the suppository 25 mg, which can be repeated, if necessary, after two hours, with a maximum of two per day. The dose of the injection is 6 mg, which can be repeated, if necessary, after one hour, also with a maximum of two per day. The injection comes with a device for easy self-administration.

What about ergot rebound headache?

The ergots, ergotamine and dihydroergotamine, are long acting and maintain vasoconstriction for at least three days, as is shown in Figure 8.9 for ergotamine. This long duration of action implies that they cannot be used frequently, probably not more often than once per week. Otherwise, their use becomes associated with a gradual increase in frequency of the headaches, sometimes to daily occurrence. This is due to the development of a vicious cycle, in which the decrease in effect of the ergot is followed by rebound vasodilation, resulting in another headache. A patient in such a rebound cycle does not respond to preventive treatment and has to be withdrawn from the offending agent. When this agent is an ergot, the withdrawal is generally associated with severe headache, nausea, and vomiting. The withdrawal lasts for one to seven days and the improvement that follows, is often dramatic[18].

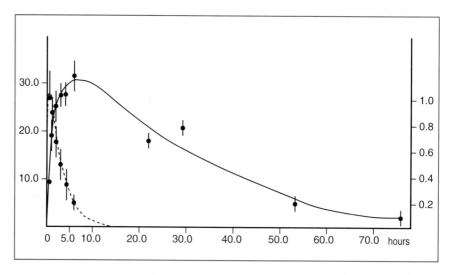

Figure 8.9. *Plasma level (interrupted line) and vasoconstrictor effect, expressed as a decrease in toe-arm systolic gradient (solid line), after intramuscular administration of 0.5 mg ergotamine. Reproduced from reference 19.*

Case study of ergotamine rebound headache

A 58-year-old man has experienced headaches since his twenties. For years the headaches occurred daily, were located across the forehead and throbbing in nature. Several times per week, they were severe in intensity. The headaches were associated with photophobia and, when severe, also with nausea and vomiting. Reading and watching television made the headaches worse, while exercise made them somewhat better. He took 1-2 mg ergotamine rectally per day for the headaches. After discontinuation of the medication, the headaches rapidly decreased in frequency and intensity. He subsequently experienced them only three or four times per month. The headaches lasted for one to three days and were mostly mild or moderate in intensity.

Case study of dihydroergotamine rebound headache

A 39-year-old woman has experienced headaches since her twenties. Initially, the headaches occurred intermittently and were mild in intensity. They lasted for several hours and were associated with lightheadedness. The headaches became daily during a period of increased stress. They were present on awaking in the morning and gradually built in intensity as the day progressed. Once every five to six days, the headaches were severe in intensity for one to two days. The severe headaches woke her up out of sleep in the early morning once or twice per month. The headaches were located on top of the head but when severe, they were located in the right or left temple, with a preference for the right. The severe headaches were sometimes associated with nausea. For the severe headaches, she injected herself intramuscularly with 0.5-1 mg dihydroergotamine. After discontinuation of the medication, the severe headaches decreased in frequency. They subsequently occurred once or twice per month, usually with menstruation and sometimes also with ovulation.

Does rebound headache also occur with the triptans?

The triptans can also cause rebound headache but only when taken very frequently. They have to be taken at least daily and probably more than once per day due to their short plasma-elimination half-lives. Exceptions may be naratriptan and frovatriptan, which have longer half-lives of six and 25 hours, respectively. The triptan withdrawal headache is as intense as that from ergot withdrawal but lasts shorter and the headaches improve faster afterwards. A diagnosis of rebound headache in general can only be made in retrospect, after withdrawal has resulted in improvement of the headaches. If after successful withdrawal improvement does not occur, rebound was obviously not present.

Case study of sumatriptan rebound headache

A 51-year-old woman has experienced headaches since her teens. The headaches occurred once or twice per week until five to six months ago, when they became daily during a bout of bowel problems. They were present, and at their worst, on awakening in the morning. The headaches woke her up out of sleep at night twice per week. They were generalized in location but worse in the temples and skull, steady in nature. The headaches were severe every day and associated with photophobia and phonophobia; in 40%, they were also associated with nausea. Fatigue made them worse and applying ice to the back of the head made them somewhat better. She took sumatriptan 6 mg by injection daily, often twice per day. The sumatriptan was discontinued and she was given a three day course of prednisone. She had a severe headache for two days, followed by a mild headache for one day. Then, the headaches became intermittent again and she had 16 days with headache during the following month. The headaches were severe on only two occasions.

CHAPTER 9

PREVENTIVE TREATMENT

When is preventive migraine treatment indicated?

Preventive treatment of migraine aims at decreasing the occurrence of the headaches. It involves the daily intake of a medication for a shorter (short-term prevention) or longer period of time (long-term prevention). Short-term prevention is used when the headaches occur at predictable times, for example, during menstruation, weekends, or stressful periods. Long-term preventive treatment is generally indicated when the headaches occur more often than three or four times per month. Additionally to be taken into consideration are the intensity and duration of the headaches, as well as the effectiveness of abortive treatment.

Preventive treatment results in a decrease in frequency and, to a lesser extent, intensity and duration of the headaches. However, with effective preventive treatment, the headaches that break through can often also be aborted more effectively. Long-term preventive treatment is generally prescribed for at least six months, after which the dose of the medication is gradually decreased. Sometimes, it is possible to maintain the improvement with a lower dose or the medication can be discontinued altogether, without relapse of the condition.

Which medications can be used for the preventive treatment of migraine?

The medications that have been shown to be effective in migraine prevention can be divided into five categories: ergots, β-adrenoceptor blockers, tricyclics, calcium-entry blockers, and anticonvulsants[3].

The ergots, dihydroergotamine, ergotamine, and methysergide, have a relatively rapid onset of action and, therefore, are best used for short-term prevention. A problem with the long-term use of methysergide in particular is the potential occurrence of fibrotic conditions[1]. Most common is retroperitoneal fibrosis, with the formation of fibrotic tissue in the retroperitoneal space. Less common are pleuropulmonary and endocardial fibrosis, with fibrotic tissue formed in the lungs and heart, respectively. Retroperitoneal fibrosis manifests itself through pain in the abdomen or back, or swelling of the legs. The pain in the abdomen or back is caused by hydronephrosis due to ureteral obstruction. The swelling of the legs is caused by obstruction of the inferior vena cava. Pleuropulmonary fibrosis manifests itself through chest pain and shortness of breath. Endocardial fibrosis generally remains asymptomatic but is characterized by the development of cardiac murmurs. Interrupting the (long-term) treatment with methysergide for four weeks every four to six months can generally prevent the occurrence of clinically significant fibrosis.

Case study of methysergide-induced retroperitoneal fibrosis

A 37-year-old woman has experienced headaches since age 17. Initially, the headaches occurred twice per year and lasted for two days. Over time, they gradually increased in frequency to two or three times per week. The headaches were present on awakening in the morning and lasted for one to two days. They were located in the right or left forehead, with a preference for the right. The headaches were always severe intensity and even worse in the week before menstruation. They were

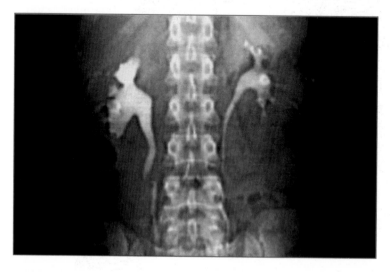

Figure 9.1. *Intravenous pyelogram showing obstruction of the right ureter at the level of the lower lumbar spine and hydronephrosis, with dilation of the proximal ureter, renal pelvis, and calices, due to methysergide-induced retroperitoneal fibrosis.*

associated with nausea and photophobia. Indomethacin by suppository and, in the week before menstruation, ergotamine/caffeine by suppository were effective in relieving the headaches. Propranolol, nadolol, and verapamil were ineffective in preventing them. However, methysergide, 2 mg at bedtime, decreased the frequency of the headaches to once every one to two weeks. She had taken it uninterruptedly for five months when she developed pain in her right lower abdomen. A pyelogram showed hydronephrosis of the right kidney, caused by retroperitoneal fibrosis (Figure 9.1).

Case study of methysergide-induced pleuropulmonary fibrosis

A 54-year-old man has experienced headaches since age 36. The headaches occurred once per week and lasted for one to two days. They were severe in intensity and associated with nausea and vomiting. The headaches were located on top of the head and throbbing in nature. They were effectively treated abortively with the ergotamine/caffeine suppository. Preventive treatment with clonidine and pizotifen was

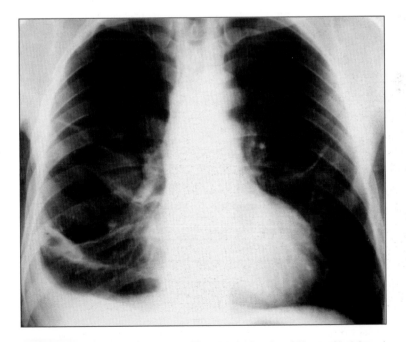

Figure 9.2. *Radiograph of the chest showing methysergide-induced fibrosis of both lungs but especially of the right lower lobe.*

unsuccessful. He was subsequently prescribed methysergide, 1 mg four times per day. After three months of taking it, he became short of breath and could no longer take deep breaths. On examination, the chest showed decreased excursion on the right and the resonance to percussion was decreased over the right lower lobe. The breathing sounds were also decreased and a crackling friction rub could be heard over the left lower lobe. Radiography showed fibrosis of both lungs but especially of the right lower lobe (Figure 9.2).

How do the preventive antimigraine medications work?

The ergots are vasoconstrictors and directly prevent the vasodilation of the migraine headache. The β-adrenoceptor blockers, effective in the preventive treatment of migraine, share a lack of partial agonist or intrinsic sympathomimetic activity (Table 9.1). This particular feature is associated with increased peripheral resistance due to an increase in vascular tone. The increased tone hampers the dilation of the extracranial arteries, thereby preventing the occurrence of migraine headaches.

The tricyclics, amitriptyline and pizotifen, potentiate the effects of serotonin through pre- and postsynaptic mechanisms, respectively. In the central nervous system, serotonin inhibits the transmission of pain signals, resulting in an increase in pain threshold. The calcium-entry blockers have also been shown to increase pain threshold[2]. This was more pronounced for nimodipine than for verapamil, which was related

Table 9.1. *Pharmacological features of the β-adrenoceptor blockers effective in migraine prevention*

	Cardioselective	Partial agonist	Membrane stabilizing	Lipid solubility
Atenolol	Yes	No	No	Low
Bisoprolol	Yes	No	No	Low
Metoprolol	Yes	No	No	Moderate
Nadolol	No	No	No	Moderate
Propranolol	No	No	Yes	High
Timolol	No	No	No	Moderate

to its higher lipid solubility. The effect of the calcium-entry blockers on pain threshold has been attributed to impairment of synaptic transmission, a calcium-dependent process. The mechanism of action of the anticonvulsant, divalproex, in migraine prevention may also relate to inhibition of central pain transmission but through potentiation of the GABA-ergic inhibitory system.

What is the best use of the preventive antimigraine medications?

Except for the ergots, the preventive antimigraine medications are best used for long-term prevention. This means that they are prescribed for at least six months, after which the dose is gradually decreased and the medication, if possible, discontinued. Long-term preventive treatment is generally indicated when migraine headaches occur more often than three or four times per month. However, as stated above, it also depends on the intensity and duration of the headaches, as well as on the effectiveness of abortive treatment.

The choice of preventive medication depends on the features of the headaches, as well as on the concomitant presence of other conditions. When the frequency of the headaches is relatively low but the intensity high, the β-adrenoceptor blockers are generally most effective. Of those, propranolol tends to have most side-effects, in particular fatigue, depression, insomnia, and impotence. These side-effects can also occur with the other β-adrenoceptor blockers but generally do so less often. When one medication out of this group fails to provide relief or cannot be tolerated, another should certainly be tried. The starting dose should be low; the dose should be gradually increased with intervals of at least one month. At the same time, side-effects, in particular fatigue, as well as blood pressure and heart rate should be carefully monitored. The β-adrenoceptor blockers are contraindicated in sinus bradycardia, atrioventricular block, congestive heart failure, obstructive pulmonary disease, including asthma, and diabetes mellitus.

When the headaches occur relatively frequently but are not so intense, the tricyclics, amitriptyline or pizotifen, are probably most effective, especially when the patient also experiences insomnia. The medications are long acting and can be taken once daily, preferably at bedtime because of sedation. Patients who do not have insomnia tend not to tolerate them well, with drowsiness on awakening in the morning. Then, a good alternative is the calcium-entry blocker, flunarizine, which can also be given once daily at bedtime. Apart from sedation, amitriptyline can cause dry mouth, constipation, and weight gain. Also pizotifen can cause weight gain and flunarizine occasionally causes depression or Parkinson syndrome. Amitriptyline is contraindicated in glaucoma, prostate hypertrophy, epilepsy, and cardiac arrhythmias; flunarizine and pizotifen do not have contraindications.

When the migraine headaches occur mostly during the night and wake the patient up out of sleep, a calcium-entry blocker like verapamil is the medication of choice. In its slow-release form, verapamil can be given twice daily; its most common side effect is constipation. Calcium-entry blockers – but not flunarizine – are contraindicated in atrioventricular block and sick-sinus syndrome because they slow down atrioventricular conduction. The anticonvulsant, divalproex, is particularly useful when mood instability is present because it also tends to be mood stabilizing. It is, however, often not very well tolerated, especially from a gastrointestinal perspective, and is teratogenic. The medication is contraindicated in liver disease or when liver function is abnormal.

The efficacy of the preventive antimigraine medications in reducing the frequency of migraine headaches is limited at 50-60%[3]. Therefore, it is important that before preventive treatment is initiated, the patient is provided with effective abortive treatment. Effective abortive treatment can, by itself, reduce the frequency of the headaches by reducing anticipatory anxiety. With regard to preventive treatment, it should always be attempted to treat the condition with a single medication first. However, if necessary, another medication can be added and a good combination is that of a β-adrenoceptor blocker with amitriptyline or pizotifen. Combinations that should be used with care are those of a β-adrenoceptor blocker with verapamil (bradycardia) or flunarizine (depression).

CHAPTER 10

TRIGGER FACTORS

What are trigger factors?

Trigger factors are events that bring on headache, the most common ones being stress/tension, fatigue, lack of sleep, and not eating on time. According to a study I conducted in my practice, more that two-thirds of patients with migraine or tension-type headache are sensitive to these triggers[23] (Table 10.1). Not only were these factors indicated almost equally frequently by both groups, they were also indicated in very much the same sequence. Therefore, they can be considered general headache triggers, independent of the type of headache, and should be mentioned to *all* patients, regardless of their diagnosis within the tension-migraine headache continuum.

Of the four most common triggers, stress/tension is generally most difficult to avoid, while the other three involve more patient control and are, therefore, easier to avoid. They result in the generally accepted recommendations that have been made to headache patients all along, namely:

1. Eat regularly during the day and don't go without food too long;

2. Go to bed on time as oversleeping in the morning – regretfully not examined in the study – is also generally detrimental to headache; and

3. Avoid excessive fatigue by pacing activities during the day and week.

In terms of their physiological impact, all four factors activate the sympathetic nervous system. Stress/tension does so through activating the ascending reticular activating system, not eating on time through causing relative hypoglycemia, which is a trigger for adrenomedullary activation, and lack of sleep, through fatigue, activates the sympathetic nervous system to boost energy metabolism. Tension-type headache typically occurs during the activation of the sympathetic nervous system while the migraine attack

Table 10.1. *Trigger factors in patients who have migraine or tension-type headache*[23]

	Migraine (n = 38)	Tension-type headache (n = 17)	P-value
Physical activity	42%	35%	
Stress/tension	84%	82%	
Fatigue	79%	65%	
Lack of sleep	74%	71%	
Specific foods/drinks	58%	35%	
Alcohol	42%	29%	
Not eating on time	82%	76%	
Cigarette smoke	61%	29%	P<0.05
Smells	61%	24%	P<0.05
Light	50%	18%	P<0.05
Noise	53%	29%	
Menstruation	57%	38%	
Weather changes	71%	35%	P<0.05

typically follows it, for example, in the evening or during the night, after a particularly stressful day (*vide infra*).

It has been suggested that patients with tension-type headache do not have peripheral mechanisms related to their pain. Instead, their headaches have been attributed to faulty pain processing in the central nervous system, resulting in a lower pain threshold. However, it is generally known that activation of the sympathetic nervous system increases the pain threshold. This would make it difficult for stress to precipitate tension-type headache if the above were true.

The migraine attack has central as well as peripheral aspects to its pathophysiology. The central aspects involve generation of the aura and lowering of the pain threshold related to the headache. Peripherally, dilation and inflammation of extracranial arteries also partake as mechanisms in the generation of the pain. The inflammation is probably secondary to the vasodilation and is neurogenic in origin, resulting from activation of perivascular nerve fibers involved in nociception. The activation of the central as well as peripheral mechanisms of the migraine attack is hampered when the activity of the sympathetic nervous system is high[22]. Reversely, their activation is facilitated on the descending limb of the activation of the sympathetic nervous system, when migraine attacks typically occur.

The specific trigger factors for migraine that were found in the study were weather changes, smells, cigarette smoke, and light. Three of them, weather, smoke, and smell, go through the nose/sinus system, if one accepts that the weather-connected headaches relate to changes in barometric pressure (*vide infra*). This would indicate a stronger involvement in migraine of the nose and sinuses than is generally considered.

With regard to the trigger factors, they generally need each other to bring on headache. Therefore, a strategy in reducing the frequency of migraine headaches is to prevent the factors from compounding. When identifying triggers, the result is that a given factor will not consistently bring on headache, which patients often find confusing.

How important is stress as a trigger factor?

Stress is a very common but not too potent a trigger of migraine headaches. In a population study, 44% of the 119 identified migraine patients indicated stress as a trigger[17]. Of the same patients, 20% indicated alcohol, 11% weather changes, and 10% dietary products as triggers. In a prospective study of 49 patients, 54% of the headaches recorded during a period of two months coincided with emotional stress[13].

Migraine headaches triggered by stress tend not to occur during the stressful event but afterwards. This was evident in a prospective study in which five patients recorded their headaches and rated five mood variables, two times per day[4]. The mood variables were nervousness, anger, alertness, happiness, and ability to concentrate. Only headache and alertness showed cyclical trends, while the other mood variables fluctuated around the zero line (Figure 10.1). The cycles of headache and alertness were out of phase with each other by one to two days, with increased alertness before and decreased alertness during the headaches. The increased alertness before the headaches could be a reflection of increased stress at that time.

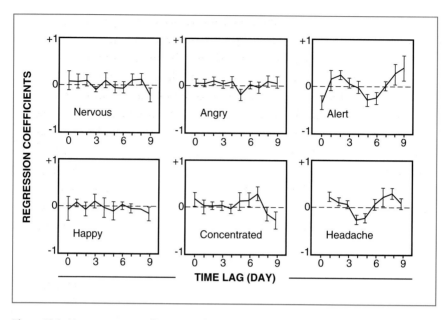

Figure 10.1. *Mean regression coefficients as a function of the time lag, in days, between measurement of the mood variables and headache, in a group of five migraine patients. Reproduced from reference 4.*

In another prospective study, 17 migraine patients recorded their headaches and ten mood variables, three times per day[12]. The ten mood variables were found to be low during headaches and the days before. However, energy and ease were particularly and consistently low on the days before headache, especially when the headache that followed was severe. This suggests that the patients felt particularly tired and constrained on days before a severe headache occurred.

My colleagues and I conducted a prospective study of 19 women with migraine, who kept a diary four times per day, at 8a.m., 1p.m., 6p.m., and 11.p.m., for 10 consecutive weeks[24]. In the diary, they recorded the occurrence as well as the features and associated symptoms of their headaches. They also rated five mood states, alertness, tension, irritability, depression, and fatigue, as well as the quality of sleep and the occurrence and stressfulness of daily hassles. They quantified the variables through the use of 100-mm visual analog scales. In the diaries, we identified 68 migraine headaches of which 23 developed during the night (34%), 19 during the morning (28%), 16 during the afternoon (23%), and 10 during the evening (15%).

The headaches that developed during the *evening* or *night* were preceded by an increased occurrence of daily hassles during the afternoon (Figure 10.2). The headaches that developed during the morning or afternoon, instead, were preceded by increased tension during the prior days. On the days before the headaches that developed during the *morning*, the occurrence of daily hassles was increased during the morning, afternoon, and evening. The increased tension at 1p.m. was followed by increased fatigue at 6p.m., which was still present at 8a.m. of the morning when the headaches developed. On the days before the headaches that developed during the *afternoon*, the increased tension at 6p.m. was followed by increased alertness at 11p.m.. The next morning, the stressfulness of the daily hassles was increased at 8a.m., followed by increased tension and irritability at 1p.m.

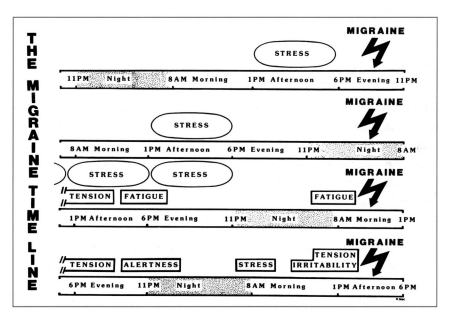

Figure 10.2. *Psychophysical precedents of the migraine attack in relation to the time of onset of the headache: the migraine time line. Reproduced from reference 23.*

The above findings suggest three different sequences of events regarding the psychophysical precedents of the migraine attack, depending on the time of onset of the headache during the evening/night, morning, or afternoon. Of migraine headaches, half apparently come on during the evening or night – for most people times of relaxation – and are preceded by stress in the afternoon. The changes in stress and mood states are more complex when the headache develops during the morning or afternoon and the simple stress-relaxation principle of migraine occurrence does not seem to apply. In both instances, there is tension at the beginning of the 24 hours preceding the occurrence of the migraine headache. When the headache develops during the following morning, the tension is compounded by stress and is followed by fatigue. The fatigue persists into the next morning – despite normal sleep – and is followed by headache in the course of the morning. It may, in actual fact, be the fatigue that brings on the headache, caused by the stress affecting the individual in a state of tension. When the tension is not compounded by stress, it is followed, after several days, by alertness in the evening, due to relaxation of the body while the mind remains aroused. The following morning, this dissociated state brings on a feeling of stress while no stress is present. The feeling of stress is extreme to the extent that it is associated with irritability, resulting in headache in the course of the afternoon.

What about weather changes?

In a prospective study of 960 migraine headaches recorded by 44 patients, the highest number of headaches was recorded on Fridays/Saturdays and the lowest on Mondays/Tuesdays[3]. The frequency of headaches was highest between September and November and lowest in February/March. The mean barometric pressure on days that headaches occurred was significantly higher than when none occurred (1012.45 mbar *versus* 1009.97 mbar; $p<0.05$). The daily frequency of migraine headaches was also higher when the barometric pressure at 6 am was higher than 1005 mbar (11.5% *versus* 8.8%). With regard to changes in barometric pressure, a decrease of more than 15 mbar over the preceding 24 hours was associated with a higher daily frequency of headaches than an increase of more than 15 mbar (11.8% *versus* 8.2%).

In a questionnaire study, 30% of 263 migraine patients indicated exposure to sun as a trigger of their headaches[25]. Exposure to sun is directly related to barometric pressure because low pressure is associated with cloudy weather (overcast). Migraine patients are sensitive to light, during and between headaches[7] (Figure 10.3), which may be why high pressure is associated with increased headache. The sensitivity of migraine headaches to decreasing pressure, as with approaching rain or snow, is well known and, as mentioned above, may indicate more involvement of the nose and sinuses in migraine than is generally considered.

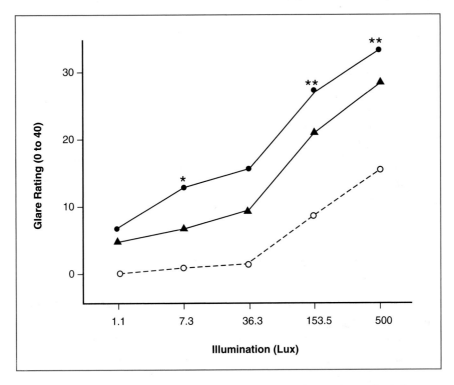

Figure 10.3. *Glare ratings in 24 migraine patients during (closed circles) and between headaches (triangles), as compared to non-headache controls (open circles; n = 20). Reproduced from reference 7.*

What about dietary products?

In a study of 490 migraine patients, 29% indicated alcohol, 19% chocolate, 18% cheese, and 11% citrus fruits as definite triggers[16]. In a questionnaire study, 1,883 women with migraine recorded all foods and drinks consumed in the 24 hours preceding headache[5]. Of the 2,313 headaches recorded, it showed consumption of cheese in 40%, chocolate in 33%, alcohol in 23%, and citrus fruits in 21%. Fasting defined as going without food for 5 hours during the day or 13 hours during the night, preceded 67% of the headaches. However, only 14% of the headaches were attributed to foods or drinks consumed in the preceding 24 hours and only 2% were attributed to fasting! In another study of 12 migraine patients, 50% developed headache after fasting for 19 hours[1].

Chocolate contains large quantities of a biogenic amine, phenylethylamine, which is a directly acting sympathomimetic that stimulates postsynaptic α-adrenoceptors[10]. It constricts the extracranial arteries and brings on migraine headache when this effect wears off and rebound vasodilation occurs. This was confirmed in a double-blind, placebo-controlled, parallel study of 20 patients, who believed that chocolate could provoke their attacks[9]. In the study, five of the 12 patients in the chocolate group developed a typical migraine attack, as compared to none of the eight patients in the placebo group (p = 0.051). The median time to onset of the migraine attack after ingestion of the 40 g chocolate given to the patients was 22 hours (range: 3.5-27 hours).

Cheese, when allowed to mature, contains large quantities of another biogenic amine, tyramine. This is a directly and indirectly acting sympathomimetic, stimulating α-adrenoceptors and releasing noradrenaline, a predominant α-adrenoceptor agonist, from the sympathetic nerve terminals. It constricts the extracranial arteries as well and causes headache by the same mechanism as phenylethylamine. However, in a double-blind, placebo-controlled, crossover study of eight migraine patients who had noticed that tyramine-containing foods could precipitate their headaches, two developed headache after 125 mg tyramine, two after placebo, and three after both[15]. In another study of similar design but involving 80 *unselected* migraine patients, eight developed headache after 200 mg of tyramine, eleven after placebo, and twelve after both[26]. The issue with these two studies may, however, be that the patients were not as carefully selected for sensitivity to the specific food trigger as in the chocolate study.

Citrus fruits contain yet another biogenic amine, octopamine, which acts as a false neurotransmitter and displaces noradrenaline from the sympathetic nerve terminals[19]. It does that in a very similar way as reserpine, which is widely reported to precipitate migraine headaches. Interestingly, tyramine is also partially metabolized by dopamine-β-hydroxylase to this false neurotransmitter.

Caffeine, also a vasoconstrictor, is present in particular in coffee (50-100 mg per 8 oz), tea (25-50 mg per 8 oz), and cola drinks

(15-25 mg per 12 oz). It brings on headache upon withdrawal, which occurs especially on weekends, partially because oversleeping delays the first cup of coffee. This was the subject of a questionnaire study of 151 consecutive migraine patients, of whom 33 (21.9%) indicated that their headaches were more likely to happen on days off and weekends than on weekdays[2]. These patients had a significantly higher daily caffeine intake than those with predominantly weekday headaches (734 mg *versus* 362 mg; p<0.0001); they also woke up on days off and weekends by an average of 1.8 hours later (range: 0.5-3 hours). Of the 55 patients who either exceeded the average daily caffeine intake of the group as a whole (151 mg) or the average delay in waking up on weekends (0.8 hours), 4% experienced weekend headaches, as opposed to 69% of the 45 patients who exceeded both. This suggests that the above observations with regard to the occurrence of weekend headache relate to the difference in caffeine intake rather than in oversleeping.

Waking up with headache was also studied in the sleep laboratory. The occurrence of headache on awakening or the development of headache within 1 hour of getting up was found to be associated with an increased sum total of sleep stages III, IV, and REM[6].

What is the relation of the estrogen cycle to migraine?

It is the estrogen cycle in women, that largely accounts for the two or three times higher prevalence of migraine in women than in men. In women with migraine, the headaches are especially likely to occur perimenstrually and with ovulation. They also tend to be particularly severe in intensity and long in duration during these times of the menstrual cycle.

In a study of 142 women with migraine who attended a migraine clinic, 24% experienced the onset of migraine in the same year or the year after menarche[8] (Figure 10.4). Of the women who were still menstruating, 14% experienced headaches only with menstruation, 12% regularly with menstruation but also at other times, 13% with some menstrual periods only, and 45% sometimes with menstruation but also at other times. There was a relationship between the occurrence of headaches during menstruation and menstrual symptoms. The menstrual symptoms considered were weight gain, resulting from fluid retention, and breast discomfort, a direct hormonal tissue effect. When both symptoms accompanied menstruation, the likelihood of headaches occurring during menstruation was 62%, as opposed to 33% when they were absent (p<0.05).

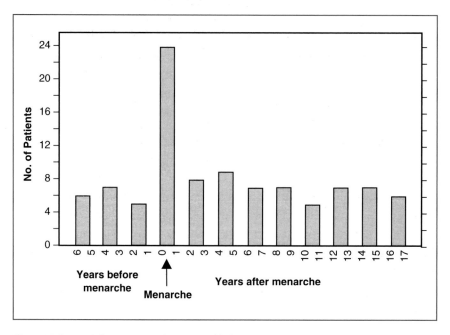

Figure 10.4. *Onset of migraine in relation to menarche in 131 women aged 14 and older, shown in years between the first headache and the onset of menstruation. Reproduced from reference 8.*

With regard to the effect of pregnancy, of the patients who experienced migraine before ever getting pregnant, 66% noted improvement, 22% no change, and 12% a worsening during at least one pregnancy[8]. Of the patients whose migraine headaches had occurred regularly and only in relation to menstruation, 90% noted improvement with pregnancy, as opposed to 38% who denied such relationship. With regard to the effect of menopause in the women who had ceased menstruating, the likelihood of improvement or worsening of migraine headaches was unpredictable, either at or after menopause.

In a study of 1,300 women who attended a headache center, in 10.7% the onset of migraine was related to menarche, in 1.3% to pregnancy, and in 4.5% occurred within 4 weeks postpartum[11]. In 2.5%, the onset of migraine was connected to taking an oral contraceptive and in 7.3%, it was during menopause. In 50.8% of the women, the headaches occurred predominantly and in 9.1%, almost exclusively perimenstrually. They were more frequently premenstrually in 56.5% and occurred with ovulation in 9.1%; 73.4% of the women also reported having premenstrual syndrome.

Of the 571 women who went through pregnancy and had migraine before that, 17.4% experienced complete relief during pregnancy, 49.9% significant improvement, 29.2% no change, and 3.5% worsening. The percentage of complete relief was significantly higher in those whose migraine began at menarche (36.4% *versus* 13.9%; p<0.001). Of the 318 women who took an oral contraceptive and had migraine before that, 66% experienced no change, 24% worsening, and 8% improvement. Of the 152 women who went through menopause and had migraine before that, 49% experienced no change, 33% worsening, and 17% improvement. Worsening of migraine after menopause was significantly more frequent with surgical than with spontaneous menopause (43% *versus* 29%; p<0.01); improvement occurred only after spontaneous menopause.

Hormonal studies in women with migraine revealed similar plasma levels of luteinizing and follicle stimulating hormones, as compared to non-headache controls[8] (Figure 10.5). However, the plasma levels of the ovarian hormones, estrogen and progesterone, were significantly higher than in the controls. With regard to the ovarian hormones, no differences were observed between the women with migraine predominantly perimenstrually and those with headaches randomly throughout the menstrual cycle.

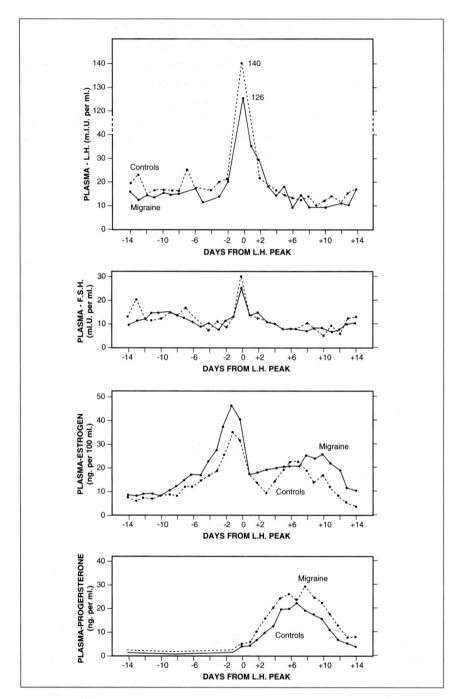

Figure 10.5. *Daily plasma levels of luteinizing hormone, follicle stimulating hormone, estrogen, and progesterone during the menstrual cycle in 14 women with migraine and 8 non-headache controls. Reproduced from reference 8.*

In relation to the changes in plasma estrogen and progesterone, the headaches in women with menstrual migraine occur during the terminal phase of estrogen and progesterone withdrawal, as is illustrated in Figure 10.6. Artificially maintaining the plasma estrogen level through administration of estradiol delayed the migraine headache, while the progesterone withdrawal and menstruation still occurred[21]. Administration of progesterone had the opposite effect: it delayed menstruation while the migraine headache still occurred[20].

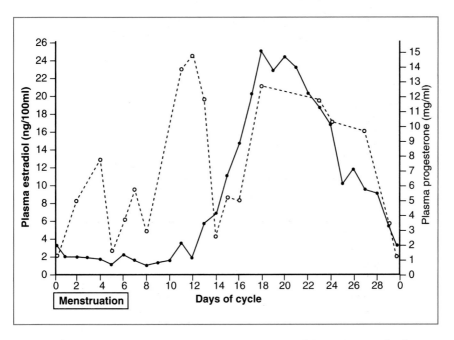

Figure 10.6. *Daily plasma estradiol and progesterone levels determined during a menstrual cycle in a woman with menstrual migraine. The arrow indicates the occurrence of the migraine headache. Reproduced from reference 20.*

What about the use of oral contraceptives?

Oral contraceptives generally contain an estrogen and progestogen. They suppress ovulation but do not eliminate or alleviate the estrogen cycle and cause more pronounced estrogen withdrawal before the monthly bleeding occurs. Therefore, it is not surprising that oral contraceptives often aggravate migraine headaches, especially when the headaches are menstrually related. This was confirmed in a randomized, open-label, crossover study of a 50-μg oral contraceptive in 40 patients with migraine[18]. The oral contraceptive was taken for two months, preceded or followed by two months of no hormonal treatment. The patients recorded the number and intensity of their headaches on diary cards. The average headache index, calculated by multiplying the number of headaches by the intensity on a 3-point scale, was 48.7 during the two months of oral-contraceptive treatment and 32.8 during the two months of no hormonal treatment. In another study of 56 migraine patients who used oral contraceptives, 70% improved after they were discontinued[14]. Of those who experienced more than four headaches per month (n = 30), 87% improved, with improvement defined as a decrease in headache frequency of at least 60%.

What about menopausal estrogen therapy?

The estrogens used most frequently for menopausal therapy are the conjugated estrogens obtained from the urine of pregnant mares, or synthetic estradiol. The medications are often given cyclically in combination with a progestogen to prevent endometrial hyperplasia. However, this is actually not necessary and the estrogen(s) can be given daily with a small dose of progestogen, or the progestogen can be given cyclically. Like migraine patients on oral contraceptives, patients on menopausal estrogen therapy have headaches more frequently. In a study, 47% of 87 patients had more than four headaches per month, as compared to 27% of 92 women who were not on hormonal treatment[14]. In a group of 78 patients on menopausal estrogen therapy, 58% improved after decycling the estrogen therapy and decreasing the dose by half or more. Improvement was again defined as a decrease in headache frequency of at least 60%.

DR. GRAHAM'S LESSONS

FOR MIGRAINE PATIENTS AND THEIR PHYSICIANS

In 1955/56, John R. Graham, M.D., M.A.C.P., published a little medical book, titled: *Treatment of Migraine**, in which he provided valuable advise for patients with migraine and for the physicians treating them.

Dr. Graham (1909-1990) first became interested in headache as a medical student at Harvard while working under F. Dennette Adams, M.D., in the Headache Clinic of the Massachusetts General Hospital, Boston, in 1934. Later, as a resident at the New York Hospital, he worked under Harold G. Wolff, M.D., and with his assistance carried out experiments, that helped to explain the action of ergotamine in relieving the pain of the migraine headache. On his return to Boston in 1937 – with the exception of the wartime – he worked in the Headache Clinic of the Massachusetts General Hospital of which he became the Director in 1946.

In 1950, he became the Chief of Medical Service at The Faulkner Hospital in Boston, where he established The Headache Research Foundation. He remained the Director of the Foundation until his retirement in 1986. The following is reproduced, with slight adaptations, from his book.

Ten commandments of migraine prevention

I. At present, there is no magic medicine or formula of treatment that universally "cures" migraine.

II. The patient is not to "blame" for having inherited the migraine trait.

III. The pain and misery of the migraine attack are very real and not "imaginary".

IV. The patient, doctor nor husband (or wife) should be intolerant, but rather all should work for better understanding of each other.

V. The patient and the family have the greater burden in therapy, and the doctor is going to act as a friendly guide rather than as a "miracle man".

*Graham, John R, Treatment of Migraine, Little Brown & Co. Boston, 1955.

VI. The whole program will require a considerable period, with frequent reviews of progress, temporary setbacks, changes of therapeutic signals and gradual re-education.

VII. The most rewarding long-term therapy will be concerned with adjusting the patient's way of living to his or her capacities, rather than with an endless round of medication.

VIII. The patient cannot be expected to make all the necessary adjustments overnight.

IX. The changes in psychological attitudes become real only through actual practice rather than through verbal instruction.

X. There is definite hope for improvement through conscientious effort by both patient and physician but any therapeutic program rarely achieves complete freedom from migraine.

Errors in living for migraineurs to heed

A. Poor meals: skimpy breakfasts and lunches and large dinners eaten in a state of fatigue.

B. Irregular hours for meals: postponing lunch for an hour may give anyone a mild headache, but may produce a bad sick headache for the patient with migraine.

C. Morning deadlines: too little time is allowed between the rising hour and the scramble for school and office.

D. Sleeping late on Saturdays, Sundays and holidays: the patient with migraine needs a good deal of sleep – but not in the morning. Conversely, getting to bed early is important, since, to date, the only real cure for fatigue is rest.

E. Lack of breaks in the day: a short rest in the morning and afternoon, regularly obtained, is helpful.

F. Overcrowded schedules: patients usually try to work in too many events in a day. They need to spread their activities more evenly several days.

G. Failure to take proper vacations.

H.   Failure to get away from their children periodically.

I.   Excessive participation in community and church activities.

J.   Overanxiety regarding preparations for guests, shopping trips and vacations.

K.   Long automobile trips: the migraine patient usually wishes to go the five hundred miles in one day and ends up with a headache.

L.   Acting a chairman (because nobody else will accept): migraine patients do not delegate work to others – they do it all themselves.

M.   Making up for lost time: as soon as the patients are over one attack, they usually rush to repair losses. Consequently, the next attack comes sooner.

N.   Suffering petty wrongs in silence until they mount to unbearable heights: it would be better to settle differences while they are small.

O.   Aiming for impossible goals and worrying when they cannot be attained.

P.   Lack of exercise.

Q.   Lack of recreation.

MIGRAINE

BIBLIOGRAPHY

Chapter 2

1. Dahlöf CGH, Dimenäs E. Migraine patients experience poorer subjective well-being/quality of life even between attacks. Cephalalgia 1995; 15: 31-36.

2. Lipton RB, Stewart WF, Cady R, *et al.* Sumatriptan for the range of headaches in migraine sufferers: results of the spectrum study. Headache 2000; 40: 783-791.

3. Messinger HB, Spierings ELH, Vincent AJP, Lebbink J. Headache and family history. Cephalalgia 1991; 11: 13-18.

4. Rasmussen BK, Jensen R, Schroll M, Olesen J. Epidemiology of headache in a general population – a prevalence study. J Clin Epidemiol 1991; 44: 1147-1157.

5. Spierings ELH, Van Hoof MJ. Fatigue and sleep in chronic headache sufferers: an age- and sex-controlled questionnaire study. Headache 1997; 37: 549-552.

Chapter 3

1. Celentano DD, Stewart WF, Lipton RB, Reed ML. Medication use and disability among migraineurs: a national probability sample survey. Headache 1992; 32: 223-228.

2. Goldstein M, Chen TC. The epidemiology of disabling headache. Adv Neurol 1982; 33: 377-390.

3. Lipton RB, Stewart WF, Diamond S, *et al.* Diamond ML, Reed M. Prevalence and burden of migraine in the United States: data from the American Migraine Study II. Headache 2001; 41: 646-657.

4. Lipton RB, Stewart WF, Celentano DD, Reed ML. Undiagnosed migraine headaches: a comparison of symptom-based and reported physician diagnosis. Arch Intern Med 1992; 152: 1273-1278.

5. Mattsson P, Svardsudd K, Lundberg PO, Westerberg CE. The prevalence of migraine in women aged 40-74 years: a population-based study. Cephalalgia 2000; 20: 893-899.

6. Rasmussen BK, Jensen R, Schroll M, Olesen J. Epidemiology of headache in a general population - a prevalence study. J Clin Epidemiol 1991; 44: 1147-1157.

7. Stewart WF, Lipton RB, Celentano DD, Reed ML. Prevalence of migraine headache in the United States. J Am Med Ass. 1992; 267: 64-60.

8. Instituut Epidemiologie. Epidemiologisch Preventief Onderzoek Zoetermeer (EPOZ): Tweede en Derde Voortgangsverslag. Rotterdam, The Netherlands: Erasmus University, 1976.

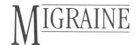

Chapter 4

1. Committee on Classification of Headache of the National Institute of Neurological Diseases and Blindness. Classification of headache. J Am Med Ass 1962; 179: 717-718.

2. Headache Classification Committee of the International Headache Society. Classification and diagnostic criteria for headache disorders, cranial neuralgias and facial pain. Cephalalgia 1988; 8 (suppl 7): 1-96.

3. Spierings ELH. Angiographic changes suggestive of vasospasm in migraine complicated by stroke. Headache 1990; 30: 727-728.

4. Milhaud D, Bogousslavsky J, Van Melle G, Liot P. Ischemic stroke and active migraine. Neurology 2001; 57: 1805-1811.

5. Spierings ELH. Flurries of migraine (with) aura and migraine aura status letter. Headache 2002; 42: 326-327.

Chapter 5

1. Ray BS, Wolff HG. Pain-sensitive structures of the head and their significance in headache. Arch Surg 1940; 41: 813-856.

2. Spierings ELH. Recent advances in the understanding of migraine. Headache 1988; 28: 655-658.

3. Vincent AJP, Spierings ELH, Messinger HB. A controlled study of visual symptoms and eyestrain factors in chronic headache. Headache 1989; 29: 523-527.

Chapter 6

1. Anselmi B, Baldi E, Casacci F, Salmon S. Endogenous opioids in cerebrospinal fluid and blood in idiopathic headache sufferers. Headache 1980; 20: 294-299.

2. Burnstein R, Yarnitsky D, Goor-Aryeh I, et al. An association between migraine and cutaneous allodynia. Ann Neurol 2000; 47: 614-624.

3. Chapman LF, Ramos AO, Goodell H, et al. A humoral agent implicated in vascular headache of the migraine type. Arch Neurol 1960; 3: 223-229.

4. De Hoon JNJM. Migraine and anti-migraine drugs. Focus on cardiovascular aspects. Thesis, University Maastricht, The Netherlands, 2000.

5. Goadsby PJ, Edvinsson L, Ekman R. Vasoactive peptide release in the extracerebral circulation of human during migraine headache. Ann Neurol 1990; 28: 183-187.

6. Graham JR, Wolff HG. Mechanism of migraine headache and action of ergotamine tartrate. Arch Neurol Psychiat 1938; 39: 737-763.

7. Hare EH. Personal observations on the spectral march of migraine. J Neurol Sci 1966; 3: 259-264.

8. Iversen HK, Nielsen TH, Olesen J, Tfelt-Hansen P. Arterial responses during migraine headache. Lancet 1990; 336: 837-839.

9. Marcussen RM, Wolff HG. 1. Effects of carbon dioxide-oxygen mixtures given during preheadache phase of the migraine attack. 2. Further analysis of the pain mechanisms in headache. Arch Neurol Psychiat 1950; 63: 42-51.

10. Milner PM. Note on a possible correspondence between the scotomas of migraine and spreading depression of Leão. Electroencephalogr Clin Neurophysiol 1958; 10: 705.

11. Olesen J, Friberg L, Olsen TS, et al. Timing and topography of cerebral blood flow, aura, and headache during migraine attacks. Ann Neurol 1990: 28: 791-798.

12. Olesen J, Larsen B, Lauritzen M. Focal hyperemia followed by spreading oligemia and impaired activation of rCBF in classic migraine. Ann Neurol 1981; 9: 344-352.

13. Ophoff RA, Terwindt GM, Vergouwe MN, et al. Familial hemiplegic migraine and episodic ataxia type-2 are caused by mutations in the Ca2+ channel gene CACNL1A4. Cell 1996; 87: 543-552.

14. Palmer JE. Chronicle EP, Rolan P, Mulleners WM. Cortical hyperexcitability is cortical under-inhibition: evidence from a novel functional test of migraine patients. Cephalalgia 2000: 20: 525-532.

15. Sanchez del Rio M, Bakker D, Wu O, et al. Perfusion weighted imaging during migraine: spontaneous visual aura and headache. Cephalalgia 1999; 19: 701-707.

16. Schumacher GA, Wolff HG. A. Contrast of histamine headache with the headache of migraine and that associated with hypertension. B. Contrast of vascular mechanisms in preheadache and in headache phenomena of migraine. Arch Neurol Psychiat 1941; 45: 199-214.

17. Spierings ELH. Recent advances in the understanding of migraine. Headache 1988; 28: 655-658.

18. Tunis MM, Wolff HG. Long-term observations of the reactivity of the cranial arteries in subjects with vascular headache of the migraine type. Arch Neurol Psychiat 1953; 70: 551-557.

19. Spierings ELH. Angiographic changes suggestive of vasospasm in migraine complicated by stroke. Headache 1990; 30: 727-728.

20. Weiller C, May A, Limmroth V, et al. Brain stem activation in spontaneous human migraine attacks. Nature Med 1995; 1: 658-660.

21. Welch KMA, Levine SR, D'Andrea G, *et al.* Preliminary observations on brain energy metabolism in migraine studied by in vivo phosphorus 31 NMR spectroscopy. Neurology 1989; 39: 538-541.

22. Wolff HG, Tunis MM, Goodell H. Evidence of tissue damage and changes in pain sensitivity in subjects with vascular headaches of the migraine type. Arch Int Med 1953; 92: 478-484.

Chapter 7

1. Spierings ELH. Differentiating headache from organic disease. Intern Med 1988; 9(10): 106-131.

2. Spierings ELH. Chronic daily headache: a review. Headache Q 2000; 11: 181-196.

3. Spierings ELH. Headache continuum: concept and supporting evidence from recent study of chronic daily headache. Clin J Pain 2001; 17: 337-340.

4. Spierings ELH, Schroevers M, Honkoop PC, Sorbi. Presentation of chronic daily headache: a clinical study. Headache 1998; 38: 191-196.

5. Spierings ELH, Schroevers M, Honkoop PC, Sorbi. Development of chronic daily headache: a clinical study. Headache 1998; 38: 529-533.

6. Spierings ELH, Ranke AH, Schroevers M, Honkoop PC. Chronic daily headache: a time perspective. Headache 2000; 40: 306-310.

Chapter 8

1. Boyle R, Behan PO, Sutton JA. A correlation between severity of migraine and delayed gastric emptying measured by an epigastric impedance method. Br J Clin Pharmacol 1990; 30: 405-409.

2. Chapman LF, Ramos AO, Goodell H, *et al.* A humoral agent implicated in vascular headache of the migraine type. Arch Neurol 1960; 3: 223-229.

3. De Hoon JNJM. Migraine and anti-migraine drugs. Focus on cardiovascular aspects. Thesis, University Maastricht, The Netherlands, 2000.

4. Goadsby PJ, Edvinsson L. Sumatriptan reverses the changes in calcitonin gene-related peptide seen in the headache phase of migraine. Cephalalgia 1991; 11 (suppl 11): 3-4.

5. Graham JR. Rectal use of ergotamine tartrate and caffeine alkaloid for the relief of migraine. N Engl J Med 1954; 250: 936-938.

6. Graham JR, Wolff HG. Mechanism of migraine headache and action of ergotamine tartrate. Arch Neurol Psychiat 1938; 39: 737-763.

7. Heyck H. Pathogenesis of migraine. Res Clin Stud Headache 1969; 2: 1-28.

8. Kaufman J, Levine I. Acute gastric dilatation of the stomach during attack of migraine. Radiology 1936; 27: 301-302.

9. Laska EM, Sunshine A, Mueller F, *et al.* Caffeine as an analgesic adjuvant. J Am Med Ass 1984; 251: 1711-1718.

10. Salonen R, Petricoul O, Sabin A, *et al.* Encapsulation delays absorption of sumatriptan tablets (abstract). Cephalalgia 2000; 20: 423-424.

11. Sheftell FD, O'Quinn S, Watson C, *et al.* Low migraine recurrence with naratriptan: clinical parameters related to recurrence. Headache 2000; 40: 103-110.

12. Spierings ELH. Treatment of the migraine attack. In: Ferrari MD, Lataste X (eds). Migraine and Other Headaches. Park Ridge, New Jersey: Parthenon, 1989: 241-247.

13. Spierings ELH. Optimum-dose determination of the triptans (abstract). Headache 2000; 40: 433-434.

14. Spierings ELH. The (suma)triptan history revisited (letter). Headache 2000; 40: 766-767.

15. Spierings ELH. Eletriptan in acute migraine: a double-blind, placebo-controlled comparison to sumatriptan (letter). Neurlogy 2000; 55: 735-736.

16. Spierings ELH, Keywood C. Clinical factors associated with low headache recurrence with frovatriptan (abstract). Cephalalgia 2000; 20: 340.

17. Spierings ELH, Saxena PR. Effect of ergotamine on cranial arteriovenous shunting in experiments with constant flow perfusion. Eur J Pharmacol 1979; 56: 31-37.

18. Tfelt-Hansen P, Aebelholt Krabbe A. Ergotamine abuse. Do patients benefit from withdrawal? Cephalalgia 1981; 1: 29-32.

19. Tfelt-Hansen P, Paalzow L. Intramuscular ergotamine: plasma levels and dynamic activity. Clin Pharmacol Ther 1985; 37: 29-35.

20. Volans GN. The effect of metoclopramide on the absorption of effervescent aspirin in migraine. Br J Clin Pharmacol 1975; 2: 57-63.

21. Waelkens J. Domperidone in the prevention of complete classical migraine. Br Med J 1982; 284: 944.

Chapter 9

1. Graham JR, Suby HI, LeCompte PM, Sadowsky NL. Inflammatory fibrosis associated with methysergide therapy. Res Clin Stud Headache 1967; 1: 123-164.

2. Miranda HF, Bustamante D, Kramer V, et al. Antinociceptive effects of Ca^{2+} channel blockers. Eur J Pharmacol 1992; 217: 137-141.

3. Spierings ELH. Management of Migraine. Boston, Massachusetts: Butterworth-Heinemann, 1996.

Chapter 10

1. Blau JN, Cumings JN. Method of precipitating and preventing some migraine attacks. Br Med J 1966; 2: 1242-1243.

2. Couturier EGM, Hering R, Steiner TJ. Weekend attacks in migraine patients: caused by caffeine withdrawal? Cephalalgia 1992; 12: 99-100.

3. Cull RE. Barometric pressure and other factors in migraine. Headache 1981; 21: 102-104.

4. Dalkvist J, Ekbom K, Waldenlind E. Headache and mood: a time-series analysis of self-ratings. Cephalalgia 1984; 4: 45-52.

5. Dalton K. Food intake prior to migraine attack - study of 2,313 spontaneous attacks. Headache 1975; 15: 188-193.

6. Dexter JD. The relationship between stages III + IV + REM sleep and arousals with migraine. Headache 1979; 19: 364-369.

7. Drummond PD. A quantitative assessment of photophobia in migraine and tension headache. Headache 1986; 26: 465-469.

8. Epstein MT, Hockaday JM, Hockaday TDR. Migraine and reproductive hormones throughout the menstrual cycle. Lancet 1975; 1: 543-548.

9. Gibb CM, Davies PTG, Glover V, et al. Chocolate is a migraine-provoking agent. Cephalalgia 1991; 11: 93-95.

10. Gonsalves A, Johnson ES. Possible mechanism of action of beta-phenylethylamine in migraine. J Pharm Pharmacol 1977; 29: 646.

11. Granella F, Sances G, Zanferrari C, et al. Migraine without aura and reproductive life events: a clinical epidemiological study in 1300 women. Headache 1993; 33: 385-389.

12. Harrigan JA, Kues JR, Ricks DF, Smith R. Moods that predict coming migraine headaches. Pain 1984; 20: 385-396.

13. Henryk-Gutt R, Rees WL. Psychological aspects of migraine. J Psychosom Res 1973; 17: 141-153.

14. Kudrow L. The relationship of headache frequency to hormone use in migraine. Headache 1975; 15: 36-40.

15. Moffett A, Swash M, Scott DF. Effect of tyramine in migraine: a double-blind study. J Neurol Neurosurg Psychiat 1972; 35: 496-499.

16. Peatfield RC, Glover V, Littlewood JT, et al. The prevalence of diet-induced migraine. Cephalalgia 1984; 4: 179-183.

17. Rasmussen BK. Migraine and tension-type headache in a general population: precipitating factors, female hormones, sleep pattern and relation to lifestyle. Pain 1993; 53: 65-72.

18. Ryan RE. A controlled study of the effect of oral contraceptives on migraine. Headache 1978; 17: 250-252.

19. Sever PS. False transmitter and migraine. Lancet 1997; 1: 333.

20. Somerville BW. The role of progesterone in menstrual migraine. Neurology 1971; 21: 853-859.

21. Somerville BW. The role of estradiol withdrawal in the etiology of menstrual migraine. Neurology 1972; 22: 355-365.

22. Spierings ELH. The physiology and biochemistry of stress in relation to headache. In: Adler CS, Adler SM, Packard RC (eds). Psychiatric Aspects of Headache. Baltimore, Maryland: Williams and Wilkins, 1987: 237-253.

23. Spierings ELH, Ranke AH, Honkoop PC. Precipitating and aggravating factors of migraine versus tension-type headache. Headache; 2001: 41: 554-558.

24. Spierings ELH, Sorbi M, Maassen GH, Honkoop PC. Psychophysical precedents of migraine in relation to the time of onset of the headache: the migraine time line. Headache 1997; 37: 217-220.

25. Vijayan N, Gould S, Watson C. Exposure to sun and precipitation of migraine. Headache 1980; 20: 42-43.

26. Ziegler DK, Stewart R. Failure of tyramine to induce migraine. Neurology 1977; 27: 725-726.

MIGRAINE